# Chagas Disease - From Cellular and Molecular Aspects of *Trypanosoma cruzi*-Host Interactions to the Clinical Intervention

*Edited by Rubem Menna-Barreto*

Published in London, United Kingdom

Chagas Disease - From Cellular and Molecular Aspects of *Trypanosoma cruzi*-Host Interactions to the Clinical Intervention
http://dx.doi.org/10.5772/intechopen.98175
Edited by Rubem Menna-Barreto

Contributors
Marcos André Vannier-Santos, Ana Márcia Suarez Fontes, Juliana Almeida-Silva, Alessandra Lifsitch Viçosa, Roberto M. Saraiva, Sandra Aurora Chavez Perez Rodrigues, Alejandro Marcel Hasslocher-Moreno, Gabriel Parreiras Estolano Da Silveira, Luciana Fernandes Portela, Jacenir R. dos Santos-Mallet, Helena Keiko Toma, Luciana Reboredo de Oliveira da Silva, Teresa Cristina Monte Gonçalves, Renato da Silva-Junior, Víctor Hugo García Orozco, Juan Enrique Villalvazo Navarro, Carlos Solar Aguirre, Carlos Manuel Ibarra Ocampo, Cásar Iván Díaz Sandoval, Diego Javier Oregel Camacho, Araceli Noriega Bucio, Carlos Alejandro Ortíz Gallegos, Flávia Oliveira Cardoso, Tânia Zaverucha Do Valle, Kátia Da Silva Calabrese, Carolina Salles Domingues, Laila Gutiérrez-Kobeh, Fiordaliso Carolina Román-Carraro, Diego Maurizio Coria-Paredes, Arturo A. Wilkins-Rodriguez, Tania C. de Araujo-Jorge, Anna Cristina C. Carvalho, Roberto R. Ferreira, Luciana R. Garzoni, Beatriz M.S. Gonzaga, Marcelo T. Holanda, Gilberto M. Sperandio Da Silva, Maria Da Gloria Bonecini-Almeida, Mauro F. F. Mediano, Anthony Man, Florencia Segal, Rubem Menna-Barreto



First published in London, United Kingdom, 2022 by IntechOpen
IntechOpen is the global imprint of INTECHOPEN LIMITED, registered in England and Wales, registration number: 11086078, 5 Princes Gate Court, London, SW7 2QJ, United Kingdom

British Library Cataloguing-in-Publication Data
A catalogue record for this book is available from the British Library

Additional hard and PDF copies can be obtained from orders@intechopen.com

Chagas Disease - From Cellular and Molecular Aspects of *Trypanosoma cruzi*-Host Interactions to the Clinical Intervention
Edited by Rubem Menna-Barreto
p. cm.
Print ISBN 978-1-80355-690-1
Online ISBN 978-1-80355-691-8
eBook (PDF) ISBN 978-1-80355-692-5

# Meet the editor

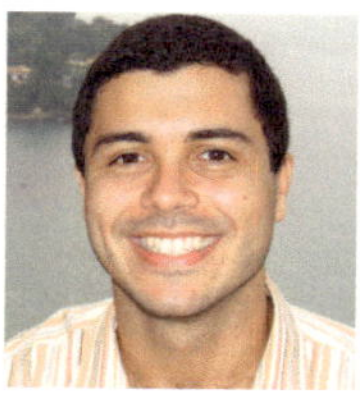

Rubem Menna-Barreto graduated in Biological Sciences from Universidade Santa Úrsula, Brazil, in 2003. He obtained a master's degree (2006) and a doctorate (2008) in Cellular and Molecular Biology, from Instituto Oswaldo Cruz (IOC), Fundação Oswaldo Cruz, in 2006 and 2008, respectively. He obtained a post-doctorate from the Institute of Medical Biochemistry, Federal University of Rio de Janeiro, Brazil, in 2010. He is currently a senior researcher at Fundação Oswaldo Cruz and a permanent advisor to the Post-Graduation Program in Cellular and Molecular Biology and Parasitic Biology, IOC. He is also a member of the Society for Redox Biology and Medicine and the Brazilian Society of Protozoology. His experience involves protozoology, chemotherapy, electron microscopy, and mitochondrial metabolism. He has published 125 papers in indexed journals and 16 book chapters.

# Contents

# Preface

Carlos Ribeiro Justiniano das Chagas (1878–1934) was a notorious Brazilian scientist, active in public health in his country. In 1909, Chagas discovered American trypanosomiasis, also called Chagas disease, an illness caused by the protozoan *Trypanosoma cruzi*. His discovery involved the description of the pathogen, the insect vector, different natural reservoirs, some mechanisms of pathogenesis, and clinical manifestations. Chagas was laureated with awards worldwide, and even today, it is considered a great injustice that he was not awarded the Nobel Prize for his discovery.

More than a century after its discovery, Chagas disease is still somewhat of a mystery. It is one of the seventeen Neglected Tropical Diseases, as determined by the World Health Organization (WHO). It affects more than 1 billion people worldwide and is endemic in 149 countries. The WHO estimates about 8 million people are infected with this protozoan, leading to 10,000 deaths per year due to complications from the disease. Since the 1990s, Chagas disease has emerged as a public health problem even in non-endemic countries, especially because of blood-related transmission (transfusion, organ transplantation, or congenital). The globalization of disease clearly demonstrates the migration of infected people from poor endemic areas in Latin America to well-developed countries in Europe and North America, among other continents. Classically, the main transmission route depends on the direct contact of humans or animals with the feces of blood-sucking triatomine insects. Infection via the oral route, in countries such as Brazil, is responsible for outbreaks of acute cases via the ingestion of food contaminated with feces or urine of infected triatomines. Serious programs must be designed to monitor the ecoepidemiology of the disease.

The progression of Chagas disease is divided into two clinical stages: acute and chronic. In the immediate stage of infection, despite the high number of trypomastigotes detected in the bloodstream, the majority of patients present with mild symptoms or nonspecific febrile illness. After a few months, the host immune system controls the dissemination of the infection, leading to undetectable parasitemia, at least by morphological methods, which characterizes the beginning of the indeterminate chronic phase. This phase is asymptomatic, usually with normal electrocardiographic and radiologic parameters. After three or four decades, one third of infected individuals progress to a symptomatic chronic phase, showing cardiac and digestive manifestations and, more rarely, polyneuropathy. The main clinical complication of the chronic stage is cardiomyopathy, determined by focal and diffuse inflammation with progressive fibrosis and electrical alterations, arrhythmia, heart failure, and secondary embolisms. The digestive form of Chagas disease involves chronic inflammation and destruction of parasympathetic neurons, culminating in the progressive enlargement of the esophagus or colon (occurring in approximately 15% of chronic patients). Molecular mechanisms related to the triggering of the progression to the symptomatic chronic stage represent the most crucial challenges in Chagas disease pathogenesis.

Reinforcing the challenges imposed by *T. cruzi* infection, up to now, the clinical treatment is still based on two nitrocompounds: benznidazole and nifurtimox, which were empirically developed in the 1970s. Both derivatives lead to a parasitological cure in almost all congenital cases (95%) and are very effective in adult acute infections (60%–80%). However, the efficacy of these drugs is drastically reduced with the progression of the chronic phase. Factors such as parasite strain and geographical area are also associated with the limited effect of these drugs, and together with their undesirable side effects, justify the continuous search for alternative treatments.

This book discusses different aspects of Chagas disease.

**Rubem Menna-Barreto**
Cell Biology Lab,
Oswaldo Cruz Institute,
FIOCRUZ,
Rio de Janeiro, Brazil

Section 1

# The State of Art

Chapter 1

# Introductory Chapter: Chagas Disease – A Multidisciplinary Old Public Health Problem

*Rubem Menna-Barreto*

## 1. Introduction: state of art

Chagas disease and its etiological agent the protozoan *Trypanosoma cruzi* (**Figure 1**) still represents an important barrier to the public health strategies, especially in Latin America, even after more than 110 years of its discovery. Tropical neglected diseases including Chagas disease have been mainly associated with low-income populations in endemic countries, but due to the globalization nowadays, an intense migratory flux is established to well-developed countries in Europe and North America, among other continents, many cases related to blood transmission (congenital, transfusional, and transplant routes) have been notified [1, 2]. It looks incredible that neglected illnesses still present unacceptable and frightening morbimortality rates in the twenty-first century. In order to change the scenario, private and special public health authorities must

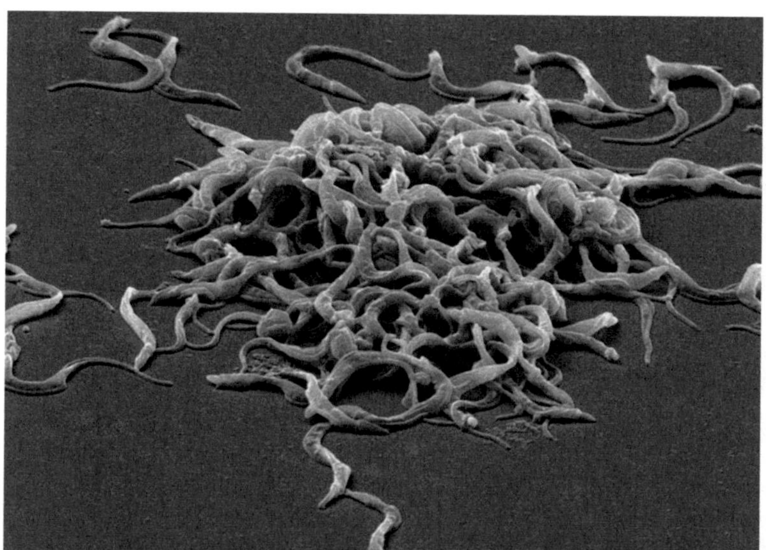

**Figure 1.**
*Countless bloodstream trypomastigotes of the protozoan parasite Trypanosoma cruzi. Micrograph produced by Drs. Helene Barbosa and RubemMenna-Barreto in Jeol JSM6390LV scanning electron microscope located in Plataforma de MicroscopiaEletrônica Rudolf Barth (Instituto Oswaldo Cruz, Fiocruz). Bar: 10 µm.*

work together, giving the veritable attention to these diseases, what would culminate in a reduction in the number of deaths [3].

## 2. The disease

Epidemiological data from World Health Organization point to 21 Latin American countries endemic of Chagas disease, estimated 6 to 7 million infected people, and 75 million under risk of infection worldwide. This illness possesses two clinical phases: acute and chronic. Patent parasitemia and intense tissue inflammation are the characteristics of acute phase, usually oligosymptomatic [4]. After few months, chronic phase starts in an indeterminate form without any clinical signs or symptoms. Almost 70% of infected individuals will not progress to the symptomatic chronic stage, remaining in this phase for the rest of their lives. The most frequent clinical manifestation observed in chronic phase is cardiac dysfunction, more severe when compared to the other cardiomyopathies, the main cause of mortality in chronic patients. Heart complications are directly associated with the high socioeconomic impact, generating expenditure in the range of billions of dollars annually, as well as the loss of productivity of affected individuals. To avoid mortality and excessive financial expense, more studies about biomarkers for early prognosis should be incited. More groups should develop applicable research focused in this area [5].

## 3. The treatment: past, present, and future

On the other hand, the treatment of Chagas disease is restricted to the use of two nitroderivatives called benznidazole and nifurtimox developed more than half century ago, presenting its effectiveness is controversial, especially in the chronic phase. Undesirable side effects together with limited efficacy among different parasite stocks justify the intense and continuous efforts to find alternative anti-*T. cruzi* compounds; however, few drugs have reached the stage of clinical trials up to now [6]. The better understanding of cellular, molecular, and biochemical mechanisms involved in the infection of vertebrate hosts, as well as essential processes in the parasite, can provide subsidies that direct for the development of more effective drugs, and which have fewer adverse effects. It is important to encourage projects and research lines in this direction.

Another no less important point is the use of non-pharmacological approaches in the patients. As an example, it is well known that physical training improves the immune response against many kinds of infections in heart tissue. Once that the worsening of the cardiac alterations in Chagas disease has been related to the prooxidant and immunological responses triggered by the parasite, strategies that promote exacerbation of anti-inflammatory and antioxidant machinery produce protective effects against tissue injury. Recently, our group described the anti-fibrotic effect of the physical exercise in indeterminate stage model in mice, suggesting that regular physical training in indeterminate individuals could partial attenuate the progression of the cardiac lesion [7]. However, further studies analyzing the correlation physical exercise and progression of heart dysfunction must be performed in near future to answer this open question. The search of alternative approaches must be stimulated, once the chronic patients today cannot wait for the development of new drugs.

## Author details

Rubem Menna-Barreto
Laboratório de BiologiaCelular, Instituto Oswaldo Cruz, Fundação Oswaldo Cruz, Rio de Janeiro, Brazil

*Address all correspondence to: rubemsadok@gmail.com

## References

[1] Coura JR, Viñas PA. Chagas disease: A new worldwide challenge. Nature. 2010;**465**(7301):S6-S7. DOI: 10.1038/nature09221

[2] World Health Organization. Chagas Disease (Also Known as American Trypanosomiasis). 2021. World Health Organization. Available from: https://www.who.int/news-room/fact-sheets/detail/chagas-disease-(americantrypanosomiasis) [Accessed: January, 2021]

[3] Menna-Barreto RFS, Santos ALS. Editorial: Molecular mechanisms of action of trypanocidal and leishmanicidal drugs with focus on novel chemotherapeutic strategies: Creation of a Brazilian multicentre working group. Memórias do Instituto Oswaldo Cruz. 2022;**117**:e220002. DOI: 10.1590/0074-02760220002

[4] Menna-Barreto RF, de Castro SL. Clear shot at primary aim: Susceptibility of *Trypanosoma cruzi* organelles, structures and molecular targets to drug treatment. Current Topics in Medicinal Chemistry. 2017;**17**(10):1212-1234. DOI: 10.2174/1568026616666161025161858

[5] Caminha MA, de Lorena VMB, de Oliveira JW, Perales J, Carvalho PC, Lima DB, et al. *Trypanosoma cruzi*immunoproteome: Calpain-like CAP5.5 differentially detected throughout distinct stages of human Chagas disease cardiomyopathy. Journal of Proteomics. 2019;**194**:179-190. DOI: 10.1016/j.jprot.2018.11.019

[6] Dantas-Pereira L, Cunha-Junior EF, Andrade-Neto VV, Bower JF, Jardim GAM, da Silva Júnior EN, et al. Naphthoquinones and derivatives for chemotherapy: Perspectives and limitations of their anti-trypanosomatids activities. Current Pharmaceutical Design. 2021;**27**(15):1807-1824. DOI: 10.2174/1381612826666201109111802

[7] Pedra-Rezende Y, Barbosa JMC, Bombaça ACS, Dantas-Pereira L, Gibaldi D, Vilar-Pereira G, et al. Physical exercise promotes a reduction in cardiac fibrosis in the chronic indeterminate form of experimental chagas disease. Frontiers in Immunology. 2021;**12**:712034. DOI: 10.3389/fimmu.2021.712034

Section 2

# The Treatment

Chapter 2

# New Therapeutics for Chagas Disease: Charting a Course to Drug Approval

*Anthony Man and Florencia Segal*

## Abstract

Little progress has been made since the 1960s and 1970s to widen the therapeutic arsenal against *Trypanosoma cruzi*, the causative pathogen of Chagas disease, which remains a frustrating and perplexing infectious disease. This chapter focuses on the strategic and operational challenges in the clinical drug development of a novel antitrypanosomal agent for Chagas disease. The various elements that contribute to a robust assessment of treatment effect including dose selection, choice of patient population, trial methodology, endpoint measures, and regulatory perspectives are discussed. The learnings herein should serve as resource to help researchers and other stakeholders optimize their clinical development plans and speed delivery of new medicines to patients with Chagas disease.

**Keywords:** Chagas disease, challenges, clinical, drug development, strategy, therapeutics, regulatory approval

## 1. Introduction

Chagas disease is a largely vector-borne infection caused by *Trypanosoma cruzi*, a kinetoplastid protozoan parasite endemic to Latin America. It affects an estimated 6–7 million people globally, is associated with 1.2 million cases of cardiomyopathy, and causes 10–14,000 deaths annually [1, 2]. While most infections are transmitted by triatomine insects, infection can be acquired through oral routes, congenital infection, and organ transplantation. For many decades, Chagas disease was mainly seen in rural populations of Central and South America, but in recent years the number of cases diagnosed in urban endemic areas and outside Latin America has increased due to economic, cultural, and migratory patterns [3, 4]. Consequently, a drug development plan for Chagas disease must consider the international regulatory perspectives and different national healthcare systems to enable faster patient access to diagnosis and treatment.

Beyond the direct clinical impact of the disease on patients, the substantial economic impact of Chagas disease on society has been estimated by Lee et al. [5]. The annual societal cost (i.e., healthcare costs plus productivity loss) of Chagas disease globally was projected at more than over 800,000 life years lost to disability (DALYs) with a financial burden exceeding USD $600 million. When projected future costs (including cardiomyopathy and heart failure) are taken into account, the economic burden of this disease reaches a staggering USD $7.19 billion per year. In contrast, global R&D funding for Chagas disease was reported as only USD $37.12 million in 2019 (representing less than 1% of R&D funding for neglected diseases in developing countries), of which 35% came from private industry [6].

Against this economic background, the substantial resources needed to develop and approve a novel drug should be noted. Novel drug development is complex and multidisciplinary with a predicted success rate to bring a new drug to approval of less than 12% [7]. Estimated fully capitalized costs range from USD $800 million to USD $2.2 billion per compound approved. Clinical trial phases of drug development account for the majority of these investments and further costs are incurred post-approval for activities such as patient registries, follow-on studies, and drug safety monitoring.

We will discuss the various strategic and operational challenges facing physicians, scientists, and clinical researchers designing drug development programs for new antitrypanosomal agents for Chagas disease. Highlighting these issues allows researchers to explore solutions that generate sound scientific evidence for cost-effective and timely drug development programs.

## 2. Current drug therapy

The two mainstays of drug therapy in adult and children with Chagas disease are benznidazole (BZN) and nifurtimox (NFX). These two nitroheterocyclic prodrugs have been in clinical use for over four decades, and their background, efficacy, and safety are well documented [8–12]. Both reduce parasitemia and cause seroreversion but with less effect as the infection becomes more established. Both drugs are genotoxic, clastogenic, and in animals, are carcinogenic. The main inconveniences associated with their use are treatment duration of several weeks, avoidance of alcohol, and the associated clinical side effects. Adverse effects commonly seen with benznidazole are hypersensitivity reactions, skin rashes, gastrointestinal intolerance, peripheral neuropathy, and bone marrow suppression [8–14]. Nifurtimox is less well tolerated and associated with more nervous system toxicity (anorexia, sleepiness) and gastrointestinal intolerance [10].

While two drugs differ in safety profile, there is little evidence to favor efficacy of one over the other although preliminary results of one small randomized study appeared to show a slight trend in favor of BZN [15]. Results from two ongoing randomized studies (NCT02369978, NCT03981523) comparing multiple BZN and NFX regimens in adults with chronic indeterminate disease may help clarify this situation.

A simplified summary of the essential strengths and weaknesses of these two pillars of Chagas disease treatment from a drug developers' perspective is give in **Table 1**.

While a 60d treatment regimen is approved for both drugs, shorter BZN regimens show encouraging data of improved tolerability without loss of short-term efficacy [16, 17]. The results of three ongoing trials are awaited with interest; the MULTIBENZ three-arm randomized phase II trial (NCT03191162) compares both low dose for 60d and high dose for 15 d against standard 60d treatment; the nonrandomized NuestroBen phase III study (NCT 04897516) compares 2 weeks to 8 weeks of BZN and uses historical controls; and the phase III BETTY trial (NCT03672487) compares 30d of low-dose BZN to 60d standard-dose BZN in women of reproductive age.

| | Benznidazole (BZN) | Nifurtimox (NFX) |
|---|---|---|
| Mechanism of action | Prodrug converted by trypanosome specific nitro reductase (TcNTR-1)to highly reactive toxic intermediates forming adducts with DNA, proteins, and small molecules | |
| Drug resistance | • Inducible *in vitro*; multifactorial mechanisms including TcNTR mutation<br>• Intrinsic drug susceptibility highly variable across parasite subtypes | |
| Formulation & regimen | • 2.5 and 100 mg oral tablets<br>• Weight-based dosing, tablet slurry for children<br>• Typically 2–3 x day x 60 days | • 30 and 120 mg oral tablets<br>• Weight-based dosing, tablet slurry for children<br>• Typically 3x day x 60 days |
| PK Characteristics | • Cmax ≈ 2–3 hours post dose<br>• elimination half-life ≈13 hours<br>• Wide tissue distribution and transplacental passage<br>• Metabolic pathways unknown | • Cmax ≈ 4 hours post dose<br>• elimination half-life ≈3 hours<br>• Wide tissue distribution and transplacental passage<br>• Metabolism via nitroreductases |
| Efficacy | • Both drugs achieve >70% parasitological cure rate in acute phase<br>• Limited efficacy in children and adults with chronic indeterminate disease (<10–35% cure as assessed by seroreversion) | |
| Safety | • Hypersensitivity reactions (inc. dermatitis in 30% of patients)<br>• Bone marrow depression<br>• Peripheral neuropathy<br>• Mutagenic and clastogenic<br>• Embryofetal toxicity risk | • Anorexia/weight loss<br>• Nausea/vomiting<br>• Psychic alterations<br>• Excitability or sleepiness<br>• Mutagenic and clastogenic<br>• Embryofetal toxicity risk |
| Drug interactions | • Alcohol, disulfiram | • Alcohol |
| Tolerability | • BZN is often preferred to NFX due to a better safety profile<br>• Tolerability better in children and acute disease<br>• Early therapy discontinuation due to side effects is common (within 19d)<br>• Discontinuation of treatment in 12–24% patients | |

*Data summarized from multiple sources and approved product labels [14, 15].*

**Table 1.**
*Simplified summary of essential product characteristics of benznidazole and nifurtimox.*

The Pan American Health Organization (PAHO) has issued guidance on the treatment and management of Chagas disease with these drugs based on critical review of available scientific evidence [18]. These comprehensive guidelines consider the both drugs to be effective in reducing short-term parasitemia but evidence is much less convincing for improving long-term clinical outcomes. Hence, there is still much room for improvement in efficacy and safety for different patient populations. Salient points of interest in these guidelines from a drug development perspective are summarized in **Table 2**.

The preclinical and development pipeline of experimental antitrypanosomal drug candidates is covered by several reviews [12, 19–21]. Only a few new drugs have reached phase II trials, notably the azoles class represented by posaconazole and fosravuconazole (E1224). Unfortunately, both failed to produce sustained

| **Use of antitrypanosomal therapy** | **Evidence-based level of certainty** | | **Conclusion** |
|---|---|---|---|
| | **Antiparasitic and serological effect** | **Impact on clinical outcomes** | |
| Acute Chagas (children and adults) and Congenital Chagas | Moderate<br>• Parasitemia clearance (75–90%)<br>• Seroreversion (50–60%) | Low<br>• Symptomatic benefit<br>• No evidence of impact on long-term outcomes | Benefit > Risk<br>Strong Recommendation |
| Adults with chronic Chagas and no organ damage | Moderate<br>• Clearance of short-term parasitemia (RR 1.44)<br>• Long term seroreversion (OR 3.32) | Low<br>• Could reduce development of heart disease (OR 0.38)<br>• Impact on mortality unknown | Benefit > Risk<br>Conditional Recommendation |
| Adults with chronic Chagas' and specific organ damage | High<br>• Parasitemia clearance (RR 1.98) | Low<br>• No impact on progression or death | Risk > Benefit<br>Not recommended |
| Seropositive girls and women of childbearing age | Moderate<br>• Decreased likelihood of vertical transmission (OR 0.07) | | Benefit > Risk<br>Strong Recommendation |
| Benznidazole vs. Nifurtimox | Moderate for both | Low for both | Benefit > Risk<br>No evidence to favor efficacy of one or other but side effect profiles differ |

[*] *Adapted from [18]: Pan American Health Organization. Guidelines for the diagnosis and treatment of Chagas' disease. Washington, D.C.: PAHO; 2019.*
*OR = Odds ratio; and RR = Relative risk.*

**Table 2.**
*Current treatment recommendations for antitrypanosomal therapy.*

parasite suppression compared with BZN [17, 22–24] and have not progressed further. Fexinidazole, a 5-nitroimidazole approved for treating Human African Trypanosomiasis (HAT), has been tested in two phase II trials of Chagas disease (NCT 02498782, NCT 03587766). Following poor tolerability in the first study [25], a second study with modified dose regimens was conducted but results have not been published. Other novel drug classes (oxaboroles, nitroimadazoles, proteosome inhibitors) being developed for other trypanosomal diseases such as leishmaniasis and HAT may also have potential to treat Chagas disease [26].

## 3. The clinical development a new therapeutic agent

A rational starting point of a new drug development program is a thorough understanding of the "patient journey," i.e., the pathway of patient experiences from contracting infection to their end outcome which includes access to the healthcare systems, diagnosis, treatment, and follow-up. Inevitably, the perspectives of multiple stakeholders (e.g., patients, caregivers, regulators, payers, policymakers) in the Chagas disease ecosystem must be integrated into program design.

Drug developers aspire to design new medicines to match a preconceived set of criteria called a "target product profile" or "TPP." This is a statement of the desired characteristics of the drug candidate and serves multiple purposes. It is a framework for generating scientific and clinical evidence to support a final product label; it guides program decision-making and facilitates dialog with regulatory authorities. The TPP may be modified during the development process based on the generated scientific data or a shift in the external environment. Characteristics of an "ideal" drug for a Chagas disease therapeutic are given in **Table 3**, and examples of TPPs have been given by Rao et al. [19] and the Drugs for Neglected Diseases initiative (DNDi) [27].

The remainder of this chapter will focus on the clinical development stage of a new drug and assumes that discovery and preclinical development stages have been completed. Readers wishing to have deeper insights into design of preclinical programs for Chagas drug candidates are referred to the comprehensive reviews by Romanha [28] and Kratz [29].

### 3.1 Target indications and choice of study populations

As patient needs lie at the core of any new drug development program, a critical strategic decision is the choice of the patient population and the projected clinical benefit. This drives a more specific TPP, determines the associated development risks, and ultimately determines the approved drug label.

The unique and complex nature of Chagas disease, characterized by varying parasitological and clinical effects at different stages of disease, has substantial implications for clinical trial study populations and the indication chosen for approval. A schema showing the possible disease intervention points and associated challenges is given in **Figure 1**.

- Active across all *T. cruzi* strains with a low level of resistance induction
- Active on replicative, non-replicative, and dormant forms
- Sustained clearance of circulating and deep tissue parasitemia
- Convenient route of administration with age-appropriate formulations
- Low level of Drug-Drug interactions (e.g., HIV/Post TX reactivation, cardiac disease)
- Shorter duration of treatment than BZN/NFX
- Clinical efficacy in all endemic regions
- Clinical efficacy in immunocompromised patients
- Affordable and adequate product stability in endemic regions
- Superior to benznidazole/ nifurtimox in across all disease stages
- Positive treatment effect on short-term endpoints (Clinical, Serology, PCR)
- Prevention or stabilization of progression to complications (e.g. cardiomyopathy)
- Better safety and tolerability than BZN/NFX in adults, children, neonates, females of childbearing potential
- Safe for use in pregnancy
- Safe in patients with cardiac complications (myocarditis, cardiomyopathy)

**Table 3.**
*Characteristics of an "ideal" antitrypanosomal drug for Chagas disease.*

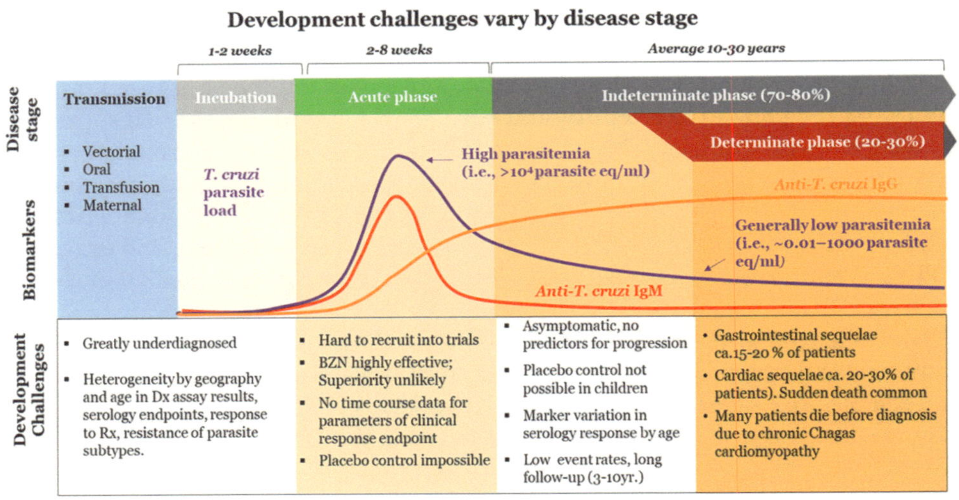


**Figure 1.**
*Development challenges vary by disease stage. (Adapted from Lidani et al. The Complement System: A Prey of Trypanosoma cruzi. Front. Microbiol., 20 April 2017).*

We will focus our principal discussion on issues associated with development in a general population of acute and chronic Chagas disease including children and adults. A pediatric development plan would be expected by most regulatory authorities. From a drug development perspective, neonates, pregnant women, and immunocompromised patients are considered special study populations and will not be further discussed in any detail. They would seldom be chosen as the first indication as the benefit-risk profile of the drug has not been fully established, but they may be included later when the appropriate supportive data are available.

### *3.1.1 Acute Chagas' disease (ACD)*

It stands to reason that early intervention in Chagas disease with an effective and safe drug, without the mutagenicity liabilities or drug interactions associated with BZN or NFX, would be beneficial. Symptomatic acute Chagas disease (ACD) is a potentially favorable setting for testing a new drug for both early efficacy and to seek an approved indication. Patients with acute disease typically have significant parasitemia and many exhibit severe clinical manifestations [30], which could serve as the basis for measurement of a treatment effect. Endpoints measures are further discussed in section 3.4.

Since BZN and NFX response rates in ACD are already high, clinical trials intended for a regulatory submission must be powered to show superiority or noninferiority and require a large sample size. In early phase II studies of a new drug, using historical BZN control data is feasible, but better is the inclusion of a concurrent BZN calibration arm to gauge assay sensitivity. A concurrent placebo control would be unacceptable in a trial of monotherapy with a new agent and rescue medication (BZN or NFX) should be offered.

The main operational challenge in ACD is the enrollment of patients for clinical trials. The number of documented ACD cases in endemic countries is low [31, 32], and even in larger countries such as Brazil, where acute Chagas disease due to oral ingestion of contaminated foodstuffs has become more common, the reported incidence is less than 0.15 cases per 100,000 of the population [33]. Prospective studies in ACD are uncommon with most published studies being case series, longitudinal cohort, or observational studies [34–36].

A modest size early phase II trial in ACD may be feasible if focused on a region of high endemicity, and a few trial sites but restricting eligibility to adults may slow recruitment rates. Interpretation of study result may also be challenging in that geographical variability in measured drug effect varies for many reasons [37, 38], and results from a small study in one region may not be reproducible in another region nor representative of a broader study population.

#### *3.1.2 Chronic indeterminate disease (CID)*

Chronic indeterminate disease (CID) is an alternative study population with both high medical need and greater prevalence than ACD. The number of studies published in chronic disease far exceed those in the acute setting and accounted for almost 80% of 109 studies in a recent review of trials in Chagas disease [36]. Patients with CID are usually asymptomatic, physically active, and have no or minimal evidence of functionally significant organ damage. As evidence for the benefit of using antiparasitic therapy in CID is not compelling, a case can be made for designing trials with concurrent placebo controls, and the CID population is becoming increasingly used for early placebo-controlled studies of experimental drugs.

Including this population in a development program is a key opportunity to prevent progression to end-organ damage and have a major public health impact. Parasite persistence is considered to play a key role in developing clinical sequelae including cardiomyopathy [39], but the pathogenesis of organ damage is not fully understood [40, 41]. Choosing cardiac-related events as study endpoints in this patient population has significant logistic challenges as event rates are low (1–2% per year), and multiyear follow-up is needed [42–44]. Even with 13 years of follow-up in patients at low risk of progression, the large randomized placebo-controlled TRAENA study of BZN (Clinicaltrials.gov-NCT02386358) failed to detect any benefit on cardiovascular outcomes despite clear evidence of an antiparasitic effect [45].

The main study methodology challenges in studying CID are choice of appropriate measures of treatment effect (parasitological, laboratory, and clinical endpoints); variability in response associated with geographical, parasitological, and immune factors; and the extended follow-up needed to establish a relationship between short-term response and long-term outcomes.

#### *3.1.3 Chronic determinate disease (CDD)*

In patients with chronic determinate disease (CDD), an antiparasitic drug might not be expected to improve established organ dysfunction, but intervention might still stop further tissue damage, worsening of cardiomyopathy and frequency of adverse cardiovascular outcomes. To address this hypothesis, a large, prospective, multicenter, controlled trial was conducted across five endemic countries. The BENEFIT study randomized over 2800 patients with Chagas cardiomyopathy to benznidazole or placebo [46]. The primary endpoint was a composite of cardiovascular mortality and morbidity events. The mean follow-up was over 5 years at the time of reporting with excellent patient retention rates. Over a 7-year period, some 60% of patients were PCR positive as baseline. and importantly these assays were standardized across reference laboratories. There was no significant difference in the clinical outcomes with primary endpoint events seen in just under 30% of patients in both arms. In PCR-positive patients, BZN causes seroreversion in two-thirds of patients compared with one-third of placebo patients. No correlation between seroreversion and clinical outcomes was seen. Additionally, the PCR seroreversion rates were much higher in Brazil than in the other countries.

While BZN therapy in CDD significantly reduces parasite load, this has not translated into significant clinical benefit. For this reason, the PAHO guidelines do not recommend antitrypanosomal therapy in this population. This trial result, however, may only hold true for benznidazole (or the same drug class) and may not predict for a new drug class with a novel mechanism of action or combination approaches.

Specific drug development challenges associated with the different populations in Chagas disease are summarized in **Table 4**.

Once the primary indication has been chosen, a cohesive set of clinical trials must be designed to generate the scientific and medical evidence to support drug registration. The foundation of the development plan will be significantly shaped by the drugs' pharmacology and its anticipated effect in humans.

### 3.2 Pharmacology and dose determination

Determining the correct dosing schedule and dosage form for a new drug is driven by basic principles of drug pharmacology. For a drug to be effective, enough biologically active substance must traverse the body's natural physiological barriers and metabolic pathways to reach the target site of action to cause the desired effect, without undesirable "off target" effects. Establishing effective and safe therapeutic doses in infectious diseases has been well served historically by pharmacokinetic and pharmacodynamic (PK/PD) modeling. This process integrates *in vitro*, *in vivo*, and human data to predict clinical efficacy and provide a rational basis for clinical regimens and trial design. The PK/PD drivers of efficacy are well recognized for many classes of antibacterials [47] and for some antiparasitics [48].

A specific drug exposure response model is assembled from preclinical data for each new compound class and validated during clinical development. All models have limitations and in the case of Chagas disease, they may be limited by the complex parasite-host relationship including differential tissue distribution, mixed infections, variable drug susceptibility, and parasite dormancy [49, 50]. Exploration of drug effects in different parasite stages, especially the intracellular amastigote form and clinical isolates from endemic regions, is recommended to support selection of a clinically effective dose. In addition, essential elements of a development program will be assessing the potential for inducing drug resistance and monitoring for resistance emergence as a cause of therapeutic failure during clinical trials. The effect on host immune response (serology) in animal models and under immunocompromised conditions provides further useful information to support clinical dosing decisions.

Sustainable duration of response is a critical success factor and the shortest possible duration of drug exposure required to obtain cure, while limiting emergence of resistance is desirable. To achieve these goals, special attention must be paid to the therapeutic index (TI), which is the quantitative relationship between drug exposure causing the desired therapeutic effect and that at which toxic develops. Animal models and PK/PD modeling simulations can provide guidance. Monitoring for recurrence in clinical trials is indispensable, and molecular

| Population | Medical need | Considerations |
|---|---|---|
| Congenital Chagas (neonates) | High antiparasitic activity better than equal to SoC<br>Prevent death, acute complications, and cardiomyopathy<br>Non-genotoxic | BZN already very effective<br>Convincing evidence of safety and long-term efficacy in older children<br>Placebo control unacceptable<br>Clean juvenile toxicology<br>Age-appropriate formulation |
| Acute disease (Adults and Children) | High antiparasitic activity better than equal to SoC<br>Short dosing regimen<br>Non-genotoxic<br>No arrhythmogenic or QT liability<br>Low DDI potential | SoC highly effective for majority of patients<br>Difficult to find/recruit patients<br>Trials must include rescue therapy<br>Placebo control unacceptable<br>Consider regions with low BZN susceptibility<br>Clean juvenile toxicology<br>Age-appropriate formulation |
| Children (early) Chronic Indeterminate | Short dosing regimen<br>Prevent cardiomyopathy<br>Less side effects and better tolerability<br>No-genotoxic molecule | Evidence of safety and prospect of benefit established in adults<br>Placebo control unacceptable<br>BZN relatively well tolerated in children<br>Clean juvenile toxicology<br>Low cardiac event rates need long follow up and large sample size<br>Age-appropriate formulation |
| Adults chronic indeterminate | Long-term seroreversion<br>Less side effects and better tolerability<br>Prevent cardiomyopathy<br>Non-genotoxic molecule | High hurdle due to long-term B-cell memory<br>BZN 30d better tolerated than 60d<br>Low cardiac event rates need long follow-up and large sample size<br>Placebo control possible |
| Adults chronic determinate | Damaged end organ rescue/ support treatments | Would a new MoA affect clinical outcomes?<br>Consider for a combination approach with antiparasitic or antiparasitic + host response modulator |
| Transplant reactivation/ immunosuppression-HIV | Effective parasite reduction as good as BZN but better tolerated<br>Low DDI liability | Patients uncommon<br>Patient polypharmacy but well supervised<br>Studies complex |
| Females of Childbearing Potential (FCBP)<br>Pregnancy | As for adults above<br>Non genotoxic<br>Safe in pregnancy | Include FCBP in acute and chronic studies with contraception<br>Clean reproductive toxicology<br>Requires extensive preclinical and clinical safety information |
| Patients with early stage I/ II cardiomyopathy | No arrhythmogenic or QT liability<br>Low DDI potential | Consider enriched population study or stratify for subpopulation in Ph III<br>Stratify for other risk CV factors<br>Large study with long follow-up needed |

**Table 4.**
*Drug development challenges associated with different Chagas disease populations.*

testing may distinguish between recurrence and new infection in hyperendemic areas. Pharmacokinetic sampling during phase II and III clinical trial is required to support dose-regimen selection, explain variability of response, and help interpret reasons of treatment failure.

### 3.3 Design of clinical trial programs

#### *3.3.1 Trial methodology considerations*

Despite the long history of clinical research in Chagas disease, the PAHO guidelines emphasize the paucity of high-quality clinical evidence. Clinical trials must be rigorously conducted, tightly controlled scientific experiments in carefully selected patient populations yet sufficiently representative and pragmatic to make the results relevant to real-world clinical practice. This balancing act is not easy to achieve and may be a contributing factor to inconsistency of trial results in Chagas disease. Trial heterogeneity is been a major confounding factor in achieving a consistent and robust conclusion on treatment effects and is evident from several systematic reviews.

A comprehensive analysis of the clinical trials landscape in Chagas disease conducted by Maguire et al. [36] analyzed 109 interventional trials of antitrypanosomal agents conducted from 1997 to 2019. One-fifth of the trials were conducted in nonendemic regions. Just over three quarters of the 23,000 patients in these studies were in active treatment arms and almost one-quarter had no therapy or placebo. Study sample sizes covered a wide range from 6 to 3703 patients with median value of 53 patients, and most studies were conducted in patients with chronic disease. Benznidazole (mainly monotherapy) accounted for 85% of active treatments and NFX for a mere 5.6%, with the remainder being azoles (2%) or unspecified drugs. These authors highlight the enormous heterogeneity of treatment regimens, study designs, and diagnostic methods and advocate a common pooled data platform to facilitate further research.

Studies addressing the impact of antitrypanosomal therapy on progression to cardiac disease were evaluated by Villar et al. [51] in their systematic review of 13 studies. Ten of these 13 studies had BZN arms, 5 included NFX, 4 allopurinol, one itraconazole, and 7 included placebo controls. Significant heterogeneity in study design, response to treatment, and patient outcomes were noted. Overall, no significant treatment effect on cardiac progression was found.

Chadalawada et al. [52] analyzed 32 trials to assess the impact of antitrypanosomal therapy on developing chronic cardiomyopathy in patients with both acute (9 studies) and chronic indeterminate (23 trials) disease. All but three of these trials were prospective cohort studies with notably heterogeneous designs. These authors found a much higher rate of cardiac progression in patients with acute disease (4.6% annually) than those with chronic disease (1.9% per annum). This increase did not appear to be influenced by the route of parasite transmission. Studies conducted in Brazil also had higher rates of cardiomyopathy than other countries. In contrast to Villar et al. this study observed lower rates of cardiomyopathy in trials with antitrypanosomal therapy compared with those without.

Patient availability may be an underlying contributing factor to the diversity of clinical trials noted above and some populations such as acute disease and pediatric patients are challenging to recruit. Identifying patients soon after infection is ideal, but unfortunately, most *Trypanosoma cruzi* infections are asymptomatic and access to diagnostics in rural areas of endemic countries is poor. While national-level screening programs may exist in antenatal/perinatal settings, blood banks, and some hospital settings such as organ transplantation, we are unaware of coordinated systematic population screening across endemic regions, which could support multinational trial participation. Most patients are diagnosed in the stages of chronic indeterminate disease (CID) or having developed chronic determinate disease (CDD) with overt clinical end organ damage. Clinical researchers should pay special attention to optimizing population screening to efficiently use study resources, time, and costs. Widening the availability and use of immunochromatographic rapid diagnostic tests [53] in endemic regions may be a useful and pragmatic approach to improved study subject screening. Furthermore, the increasing trend toward decentralizing studies and use of remote technologies [54] may facilitate participation of patients in more remote regions, especially for screening and follow-up visits.

### *3.3.2 Phase I trials*

Phase I first-in-human (FIH) studies are typically done in healthy adult volunteers. The dosing regimen, the initial human starting dose, and dose escalation scheme will be based on preclinical efficacy and adequate safety margin considerations. The usual aim is to establish either a maximum tolerated dose or a minimum biologically active dose. A comprehensive outline of the framework and general considerations for the design of FIH studies is provided by Shen et al. [55]. Although initial testing of novel drug candidates has also been conducted in seropositive patients with HIV, HBV, and HCV, this has rarely been done in Chagas disease. As of December 2021, several phase I studies in patients with Chagas disease for formulation bioequivalence, drug interactions, or drug repurposing were listed in the WHO International Clinical Trials Registry Platform (ICTRP) [56] and ClinicalTrials.gov database [57], but no FIH studies were found. Given the need to establish new and robust pharmacodynamic markers, opportunities to conduct FIH studies in populations of chronic indeterminate disease may be considered.

### *3.3.3 Phase II trials*

The first test of therapeutic efficacy where both antimicrobial and clinical effects can be measured is traditionally a phase II study (also termed a "Proof -of- Concept" or PoC) in patients with well-defined disease characteristics. The dosing regimen chosen in these studies is derived from the preclinical animal data, PK/PD modeling, and results of phase I studies. A dose close to the maximum tolerated dose seen in phase I studies may be chosen with provision for modification if significant tolerability or safety issues occur. The initial PoC study population is usually adults because only limited amount of human safety information is available. Pediatric patients are typically included later after safety has been documented in juvenile preclinical toxicology studies and in adult clinical trials.

Sample sizes in PoC studies are usually limited though efficient designs with multiple parallel arms for regimen comparison and combination therapy have become more common.

Two pairs of published phase II trials that merit further discussion illustrate some of the methodological issues for PoC and dose finding. Features common across these four studies are a multicenter, multiarm, randomized, parallel group design; enrollment of RT-PCR-positive patients with chronic (mainly indeterminate) disease; use of serial short- and long-term biomarker measurements; and PK sampling for drug exposure.

The CHAGAZOL trial [22] was an open-label, multicenter randomized trial of 79 adults conducted in a Spain comparing high and low doses of posaconazole (POZ) to 60d of standard BZN. The subject screen failure rate for study entry was 57%, and most patients (> 90%) originated from Bolivia. Sixty-five percent of subjects had chronic indeterminate disease (CID), and the remainder had some evidence of end-organ damage, primarily cardiac (22%). Serial RT-PCR measures showed a high PCR reversion in all arms during the treatment period, but by 10 months post treatment, more than 80% of POZ-treated patients relapsed versus 38% of BZN patients. The transient effectiveness of POZ in this study prompted exploration in a combination study with BZN. The STOP-CHAGAS trial [23] was a multinational study of 120 adults with CID. This partially blinded study randomized patients across four arms comprising POZ alone, BZN plus placebo, BZN plus POZ, and placebo. The higher screen failure rate of 70% may reflect the narrower patient population and broader site participation. The primary outcome measure was RT-PCR negativity at 180d. High response rates (>90%) were seen in the three active arms during treatment but was not sustained for POZ monotherapy with only 13% response at d180 compared with >80% for the BZN arms. Notably, the treatment discontinuation rate is 32% almost halving the per protocol population in the BZN arms.

The second pair of randomized studies are the trials of fosravuconazole (E1224). The single-blind, five-arm trial from the E1224 study group [24] allocated 231 adults with CID to low, high, or short doses of E1224 or to BZN or placebo. This study was conducted in two sites in Bolivia and had screen failure rate of 59% and the antiparasitic effect was assessed through serial RT-PCR and serology. The study was powered to show superiority over placebo for a primary endpoint of sustained PCR response at 12 months after treatment start. The high initial response observed for both E1224 and BZN during treatment was only sustained in BZN-treated group. The follow-on BENDITA trial [17] was a seven-arm, double-blind, double dummy study in 210 adults with CID conducted in three regions of Bolivia. Of the 518 patients screened, 210 were eligible and randomized to one of three BZN treatment arms (2,4, or 8 weeks), one of two BZN plus E1224 combination arms, or to placebo. The primary efficacy endpoint was sustained parasite clearance at 6 months based on RT-PCR. This trial showed that 2 weeks of BZN therapy was almost as good as standard therapy in achieving sustained response with far better tolerability. Whether a 2-week regimen can translate into longer-term benefit remains to be seen. The addition of E1224 to BZN did not improve efficacy but increased the incidence severe adverse events. The low rates of protocol violation and treatment discontinuation in these two trials attest to the quality of the design and execution of the study investigators.

These well-designed and well-executed phase II designs using RT-PCR in patients with CID provided a robust evaluation of drug effect and assist dose selection. This same design approach has also been used in the studies of fexinidazole (NCT02498782, NCT03587766).

### *3.3.4 Phase III trials*

The enormous heterogeneity in published studies conducted in Chagas discussed above emphasizes the need to have robust and consistent approaches to clinical testing. Typically, data from one or more adequately conducted randomized trial would be expected by regulatory authorities to support license approval. The clinical research gold standard for generating evidence of efficacy and safety is a prospective (ideally double blind) randomized clinical trial against the current standard-of-care (SoC) or placebo. In the majority of Chagas' settings, either benznidazole or nifurtimox would be the active comparative control in registration enabling clinical studies. In certain circumstances, a historical or concurrent placebo may be acceptable. The evolution of potentially shorter BZN regimens from four ongoing trials

(NCT03191162, NCT03981523, NCT04897516, NCT03672487) may significantly impact both a new drug TPP and the design of future comparative trials.

Beyond the fundamental requirements for minimizing bias and variability through randomization, blinding, and stratification, the numerous possibilities for comparative phase III and adaptive study designs will not be covered here as they must be tailored to answer the precise clinical research question of interest. The logistic challenges around designing and executing such trials to meet current regulatory standards are significant and a major investment in research time, finances, and resources. It behooves drug developers to have compelling phase II data before deciding to embark on such studies and to engage in early discussions with regulatory authorities.

A clinically meaningful endpoint (or an acceptable surrogate marker) should have been chosen and agreed with Health Regulatory Authorities; a dose adequately determined; and a minimum follow-up period of 12 months (or more) planned. Ideally, a trial should be prospective, multicenter, multiregion randomized, double-blind (double dummy), and powered at a minimum for noninferiority against the SoC (BZN/NFX) and superiority against placebo (where used). Factors known to influence variability in response such as age and geographical distribution required careful balancing. Preplanned interim analyses with early stopping rules may be useful to manage risk, and an independent data safety monitoring board is strongly recommended. Adjudication committees for some endpoints may be added as needed. Centralized laboratory assessment for serology and biomarkers is recommended.

The operational challenges of mounting large phase III interventional studies in Chagas disease include effective community engagement; cooperation with local centers of expertise; engagement of government health screening and awareness programs; rapid diagnostics and facilitated access to medical facilities capable of conducting regulatory standard studies. Rigorous trial execution and patient retention are needed to minimize protocol deviations that could compromise the noninferiority designs. Post-approval requirements may include further clinical trials or extended follow-up (3+ years) of study patients.

Where more than one drug candidate exists, prioritization decisions must be made as the resource requirements to run several simultaneous phase III programs may well be prohibitive. Clinical trial designs (master protocols) to improve efficiency of testing of multiple drugs of the same therapeutic class are well accepted by Health Authorities and have been used in oncology and more recently COVID-19 settings [58, 59]. An alternative strategic option would be a combination approach with two new drugs (antiparasitic or antiparasitic plus host response modulator) in a single phase II/III program.

#### *3.3.5 Alternative development strategies*

Discussion of drug development for Chagas disease would not be complete without considering the many outstanding strategic questions concerning the ultimate goal of halting disease progression.

After four decades of use, is it realistic to expect any more gains from BZN (or NFX) alone or is the problem simply related to poor tissue targeting [60]? Is chronic indeterminate disease already too late a setting to influence the course of the disease for any drug and if so, should efforts be redirected to early detection and acute disease where the risk of cardiomyopathy is higher [52]? Finally, would combinations of antiparasitic drugs with or without anti-inflammatory/immune-modifying drugs in both ACD and CID be more effective than monotherapy? Combination antimicrobial therapy is well established in some infectious diseases (e.g., HIV, HCV, Tuberculosis) but relatively uncommon in Chagas disease. A phase I/II trial (ICTRP REBEC-RBR-5n4htp) studying the combination of BZN and disulfiram antitrypanosomal agents is currently underway in Brazil [61]. While immunomodulatory approaches to Chagas cardiomyopathy have met with some success in preclinical models [41], there are few human trials of antiparasitic and immunomodulatory combinations. Simvastatin combined with BZN was shown to reduce cardiac inflammation in a murine model despite parasite persistence [62], and the ongoing ATOCHA trial (NCT04984616) is evaluating the effects of atorvastatin combined with BZN or NFX with chronic indeterminate disease. In a murine model, attenuated cardiac dysfunction and tissue parasite clearance were seen with the combination of fenofibrate (a peroxisome proliferator-activated receptor ligand) and BZN [63], but no human study of this combination has been published. The poor progress with monotherapy in many settings warrants preclinical and clinical exploration of combination approaches despite the potential for increased costs, more side effects, drug interactions, and increased risk of medication nonadherence.

### 3.4 Endpoint considerations in clinical trials

The scientific soundness and clinical relevance of an interventional trial are heavily dependent of choice of a robust, reproducible, and validated measurement of the desired treatment effect. Some issues related to selection of trial endpoints have been discussed briefly in the context of patient population.

#### *3.4.1 Parasitological, serological, and clinical endpoints*

Sustained decrease in parasitemia and resolution of clinical effects would be appropriate clinical trial endpoints for efficacy in patients with acute Chagas disease. Well-established microscopy-based methods exist to directly observe detection of circulating parasites; however, these methods lack the exquisite sensitivity and quantitative advantages of PCR for monitoring treatment effect [64]. Use of standardized PCR and serology assays using central laboratories is advisable during phase II and III trials to ensure consistency and comparability. Detailed time course profiles of quantitative changes in parasitemia from presentation to resolution (with and without treatment) are not available in the literature and would need to be generated *de novo*.

While a parasitological response alone may be sufficient to determine drug activity from a mechanistic viewpoint, clinically meaningful trial endpoints that reflect how a patient feels, functions, or survives are essential. Elegant and detailed descriptions of the clinical course of acute disease can be found in the literature [34, 35, 65, 66] but lack the granularity required to develop a robust clinical endpoint for regulatory purposes. If needed, additional data that enhance understanding of clinical parameters in acute disease may be sought through patient chart review (preferably from recent datasets) or by prospective collection, in parallel to, or as part of a Proof-of-Concept trial.

As, patients with CID are asymptomatic and parasitemia is often absent or of low-grade intermittent nature, most phase II studies have employed PCR testing and serological tests as to quantitate drug effects. Long-term seroreversion of *T. cruzi* specific IgG, measured by serial assays, is the mostly widely accepted evidence of cure and reflects both parasite and host response [67, 68]. PCR is considered a sensitive tool to assess peripheral parasite load for diagnosis and relapse [69] and is useful as a short-term endpoint for antiparasitic drug effect and dose finding in clinical trials [70]. Nonconventional serological tests with antibodies against specific Chagas' antigens [71] may show earlier time course changes and some (e.g., F29- ELISA, AT-ELISA) have been included in regulatory submissions for benznidazole and nifurtimox [72–74].

Some specific challenges associated with choosing cardiac related endpoints have been discussed above in Section 3.1.2 and 3.1.3 will not be repeated. Trials using cardiovascular event endpoints must also be designed to adjust for the other competing risk factors that may confound interpretation of the results [75]. Based on available evidence, the probability to detect meaningful changes in clinical cardiac parameters in studies with BZN monotherapy is extremely low. Finding new biomarkers or imaging tools that may correlate with clinical outcomes or predict for risk of later end-organ damage would significantly accelerate the development of new drugs.

The efficiency of clinical trials in Chagas disease could also be improved if study populations could be enriched by patients most likely to develop progression. Currently, no such early predictive markers of long-term seroreversion or cure exist although many markers of disease progression are under exploration. The ideal characteristic for biomarkers along with a summary of numerous parasitic, molecular, cellular, and host biomarkers studied to date has been reviewed by Pinazo et al. [67].

#### *3.4.2 Quality-of-life (QoL) measures*

Most drug studies in Chagas disease have reported adverse events or clinical effects as patient-related outcomes [36]. Quality-of-life (QoL) research using different validated tools has mainly been studied in patients with cardiac disease [76, 77]. In CID patients, QoL measures observed during treatment may be a worthwhile consideration when comparing tolerability or convenience of two active treatments. Regulatory authorities have an active interest in how patient feels and functions, and the United States Food and Drug administration (US FDA) held a patient workshop for Chagas disease that highlighted emotional, financial, and other pragmatic concerns associated with the disease [78]. Where it is appropriate to measure QoL during new therapeutic interventions, carefully constructed patient measures are useful supplements to conventional safety and efficacy parameters.

## 4. Regulatory health authority perspectives

While the epicenter of the burden of Chagas disease continues to be Latin America, migration and other factors have made the disease a global health concern. As such an international regulatory approach to drug approval is required. Early engagement with regulatory authorities in endemic regions of Central and South America is essential when designing a development program to address Chagas disease. Indeed, there is a compelling case for a single pan-Latin American approach to the evaluation and approval to accelerate patient access to new anti-*T. cruzi* therapeutics.

Outside Latin America, the US FDA has played an important role in stimulating research and development for neglected tropical diseases through several mechanisms, most notably the award of transferable priority review vouchers to eligible products and the use of expedited approval programs [79, 80]. While available in

- Serology indicates total body parasite burden and sustained seroreversion of ELISA/IIF/IHA at 3 or more years remain the standard for cure
- Serology is acceptable as a surrogate endpoint in chronic indeterminate disease
- Clearance of parasitemia alone probably insufficient for efficacy assessment
- PCR assays are an acceptable marker of failure or relapse
- Nonconventional serologic assays or PCR is acceptable as supportive evidence if multiple concordances shown with conventional tests
- Historical control data from placebo/untreated patients may be acceptable
- Efficacy demonstrated across multiple endemic regions is desirable
- Prospective randomized trials are essential because of response heterogeneity

**Table 5.**
*Considerations for clinical programs to support drug approval in chronic indeterminate Chagas disease.*

Latin America for decades, benznidazole and nifurtimox were only approved in the United States (for the treatment of children with Chagas disease) in 2017 and 2020, respectively. These drugs were assigned US FDA Orphan Drug status, and both were granted an accelerated approval based upon randomized clinical trials in children with primarily indeterminate disease using serology as the primary endpoint. Post-approval requirements (PMR) included phase IV studies to confirm activity and complete missing data gaps. As these drugs may serve as the SoC comparator in pivotal trials of a new therapy, review of the FDA assessment reports [72–74] provides useful insights into how a rigorous health authority viewed the challenges of developing a drug to treat Chagas disease.

Similar to the US FDA, the European Medicines Agency (EMA) can also grant Orphan Drug designation [81]. Furthermore, the EMA can support faster approval in certain non-European lower-income countries by providing a thorough scientific assessment and the facilitating WHO prequalification under their EU-4Mall (formerly called "Article 58") program [82]. Medicines reviewed under this provision benefit from scientific advice, EMA's PRIME (PRIority MEdicines) scheme [83], and accelerated review [84].

The authors did not find any regulatory assessment documents for indications of congenital and acute Chagas disease in the public domain. A summary of regulatory considerations linked with a clinical development program for an antitrypanosomal drug for use in chronic indeterminate Chagas disease is given in **Table 5**.

## 5. Conclusions

The development of a new antiparasitic agent against *T. cruzi* to improve the lives of patients with Chagas disease is an urgent priority and one of the most challenging in infectious diseases. Despite the discovery of the disease over a century ago, substantial knowledge gaps persist in disease biology and the pathophysiology of disease progression. Clinical trials face a wide range of challenges that include disease and response heterogeneity and operational challenges associated with early diagnosis, patient access, intervention, and prolonged follow-up. The clinical impact of the benznidazole and nifurtimox in chronic disease settings has been disappointing, but decades of research provide valuable insights that can be applied to new drug development. This discourse highlights the Chagas disease associated pitfalls to be navigated and risks that need to be managed. Ultimately, achieving improved patient outcomes requires a multidisciplinary approach encompassing novel compound classes, rapid diagnostics, early progression biomarkers, rigorous drug candidate selection, and efficient, focused clinical development plans. The advent of new digital technologies and trial methodologies has significant potential to improve clinical trial efficiency and patient access. The WHO, PAHO, Mundo Sano, the Oswaldo Cruz Foundation (FIOCRUZ), Chagas' Coalition, the Barcelona Institute for Global Health (ISGlobal), DNDi, and various private sector companies are among the many international institutions dedicated to conquering this disease. The long and complex path to the approval of new drugs will best be served by broad, long-term collaborative engagement, knowledge sharing, and partnerships between stakeholders in private and public sectors.

## Acknowledgements

The authors would like to acknowledge insights contributed by our colleagues Jonathan Spector, Caroline Demacq, Monica Quijano, and Claudio Gimpelewicz.

## Conflict of interest

The authors were employees of Novartis at the time of writing. All views are expressed by the authors to support further dialog between researchers in Chagas Disease. The opinions are not intended to represent the position of the Novartis company nor are promotional in nature.

## List of abbreviations

| | |
|---|---|
| ACD | Acute Chagas' disease |
| BZN | Benznidazole |
| CDD | Chronic determinate disease |
| CID | Chronic indeterminate disease |
| DALY | Disease-adjusted life year |
| DDI | Drug-drug interaction |
| DNDi | Drugs for neglected disease initiative |
| DTU | Discrete typing units |
| ECG | Electrocardiogram |
| ELISA | Enzyme-linked immunosorbent assay |
| EMA | Europe Medicines Agency |
| FCBP | Females of childbearing potential |
| FDA | Food and Drugs Administration |
| FIH | First-in-human |
| HAT | Human African Trypanosomiasis |
| HIV | Human immunodeficiency virus |
| HBV | Hepatitis B virus |
| ICTRP | International Clinical Trial Registry Platform |
| IHA | Indirect hemagglutination assay |
| IIF | Indirect immunofluorescence assay |

| | |
|---|---|
| MoA | Mechanism of action |
| NFX | Nifurtimox |
| PAHO | Pan American Health Organization |
| PCR | Polymerase chain reaction |
| POZ | Posaconazole |
| PMR | Post-marketing requirement |
| QOL | Quality of life |
| R&D | Research and development |
| SoC | Standard of care |
| TcNTR | *Trypanosome cruzi* mitochondrial nitroreductase |
| TI | Therapeutic index |
| TPP | Target product profile |
| TX | Transplantation |

## Author details

Anthony Man[1]* and Florencia Segal[2]

1 Global Health Development Unit, Novartis Pharma AG, Basel, Switzerland

2 Translational Medicine, Novartis Institutes for BioMedical Research, Cambridge, MA, USA

*Address all correspondence to: manyl4123@yahoo.com

## References

[1] Chagas' disease (Also Known as American Trypanosomiasis). WHO Fact Sheets. 2021. Available from: https://www.who.int/news-room/fact-sheets/detail/Chagas'-disease-(american-trypanosomiasis)

[2] Echeverria LE, Marcus M, Novick G, et al. WHF IASC roadmap on Chagas' disease. Global Heart. 2020;**15**(1):26

[3] Requena-Méndez A, Aldasoro E, de Lazzari E, et al. Prevalence of Chagas' disease in Latin-American migrants living in Europe: A systematic review and Meta-analysis. PLoS Neglected Tropical Diseases. 2015;**9**(2):e0003540

[4] Pérez-Molina JA, Norman N, López-Vélez R. Chagas' disease in non-endemic countries: Epidemiology, clinical presentation and treatment. Current Infectious Disease Reports. 2012;**14**:263-274

[5] Lee BY, Bacon KM, Bottazzi ME, et al. Global economic burden of Chagas' disease: A computational simulation model. The Lancet Infectious Diseases. 2013;**13**:342-348

[6] Chapman N, Doubell A, Tuttle A, et al. Neglected Disease Research And Development: Where To Now? G-Finder Annual Report 2020. Policy Cares Research (AU). 2021. Available from: https://policy-cures-website-assets.s3.ap-southeast-2.amazonaws.com/wp-content/uploads/2021/04/15055816/G-FINDER-2020_Final-Report.pdf

[7] Di Masi JA, Graboski HG, Hansen RW. Innovation in the pharmaceutical industry: New estimates of R&D costs. Journal of Health Economics. 2016;**47**:20-33

[8] Galván IL, Julio Alonso-Padilla J, Cortés-Serra N, et al. Benznidazole for the treatment of Chagas disease. Expert Review of Anti-Infective Therapy. 2021;**19**(5):547-556. DOI: 10.1080/14787210.2021.1834849

[9] Castro JA, de Mecca MM, Bartel LC. Toxic side effects of drugs used to treat Chagas' disease (American trypanosomiasis). Human & Experimental Toxicology. 2006;**25**(8):471-479

[10] Jackson Y, Wyssa B, Chappuis F. Tolerance to nifurtimox and benznidazole in adult patients with chronic Chagas' disease. The Journal of Antimicrobial Chemotherapy. 2020;**75**:690-696

[11] Coura JR, de Castro SL. A critical review on Chagas disease chemotherapy. Memórias do Instituto Oswaldo Cruz. 2002;**97**(1):3-24

[12] Sales PA Jr, Molina I, Murta SMF, et al. Experimental and clinical treatment of Chagas disease: A review. The American Journal of Tropical Medicine and Hygiene. 2017;**97**(5):1289-1303

[13] Benznidazole Tablets for Oral Use. Full Prescribing Information. 2017. Available from: https://www.accessdata.fda.gov/drugsatfda_docs/label/2017/209570lbl.pdf

[14] LAMPIT (Nifurtimox) Tablets, for Oral Use. Full Prescribing Information. 2017. Available from: https://www.accessdata.fda.gov/drugsatfda_docs/label/2020/213464s000lbl.pdf

[15] Coura JR, de Abreu LL, Willcox H, Petana W. Comparative controlled study on the use of benznidazole, nifurtimox and placebo, in the chronic form of Chagas' disease, in a field area with interrupted transmission. Revista

da Sociedade Brasileira de Medicina Tropical. 1997;**30**(2):139-144 (Paper in Portuguese)

[16] Álvarez MG, Ramírez JC, Bertocchi G, et al. New scheme of intermittent benznidazole administration in patients chronically infected with Trypanosoma cruzi: Clinical, parasitological, and serological assessment after three years of follow-up. Antimicrobial Agents and Chemotherapy. 2020;**64**:e00439-e00420

[17] Torrico F, Gascón J, Barreira F, et al. New regimens of benznidazole monotherapy and in combination with fosravuconazole for treatment of Chagas' disease [BENDITA]: A phase 2, double-blind, randomised trial. The Lancet Infectious Diseases. 2021;**21**:1129-1140

[18] Pan American Health Organization. Guidelines for the Diagnosis and Treatment of Chagas' Disease. Washington, D.C.: PAHO; 2019 Available from: https://iris.paho.org/bitstream/handle/10665.2/49653/9789275120439_eng.pdf?sequence=6&isAllowed=y

[19] Rao S, Barrett M, Dranoff G, et al. Drug discovery for Kinetoplastid diseases: Future directions. ACS Infectious Diseases. 2019;**5**(2):152-157

[20] Ribeiro V, Dias N, Taís P, et al. Current trends in the pharmacological management of Chagas' disease. International Journal for Parasitology: Drugs and Drug Resistance. 2020;**2**:7-17

[21] Martínez-Peinado N, Cortes-Serra N, Losada-Galvan I, et al. Emerging agents for the treatment of Chagas disease: What is in the preclinical and clinical development pipeline? Expert Opinion on Investigational Drugs. 2020;**29**(9):947-959. DOI: 10.1080/13543784.2020.1793955

[22] Molina I, Gómez i Prat M, Salvador F, et al. Randomized trial of posaconazole and benznidazole for chronic Chagas' disease. New England Journal of Medicine. 2014;**370**:1899-1908

[23] Morillo CA, Waskin H, Sosa-Estani S, et al. Benznidazole and Posaconazole in eliminating parasites in Asymptomatic T. cruzi carriers. The STOP-CHAGAS' trial. Journal of the American College of Cardiology. 2017;**69**(8):939-947

[24] Torrico F, Gascon J, Ortiz L, et al. Treatment of adult chronic indeterminate Chagas disease with benznidazole and three E1224 dosing regimens: A proof-of-concept, randomized, placebo-controlled trial. The Lancet Infectious Diseases. 2018;**18**:419-430

[25] DNDi fexinidazole for Chagas Disease. 2020. Available from: https://dndi.org/research-development/portfolio/fexinidazole-chagas

[26] Drugs for Neglected Diseases Initiative, R&D Portfolio. 2021. Available from https://dndi.org/wp-content/uploads/2021/12/DNDi-RD-Portfolio-December-2021.pdf

[27] Target Product Profile for Chagas Disease. Available from: https://dndi.org/diseases/Chagas'/target-product-profile/

[28] Romanha AJ, Castro SL, Soeiro M dN, et al. In vitro and in vivo experimental models for drug screening. Memorias do Instituto Oswaldo Cruz. 2010;**105**(2):233-238

[29] Kratz JM, Gonçalves KR, Romera LMD, et al. The translational challenge in Chagas disease drug development. Memorias do Instituto Oswaldo Cruz. 2021;**116**:1-11

[30] Bastos C, Aras R, Mota G, et al. Clinical outcomes of thirteen patients

with acute Chagas' disease acquired through Oral transmission from two urban outbreaks in northeastern Brazil. PLoS Neglected Tropical Diseases. 2010;**4**(6):e711

[31] Andrade DV, Gollob KJ, Dutra WO. Acute Chagas' disease: New global challenges for an old neglected disease. PLoS Neglected Tropical Diseases. 2014;**8**(7):e3010

[32] Chagas' disease in Latin America: An epidemiological update based on 2010 estimates. Weekly Epidemiological Record. 2015;**90**(6):33-43

[33] Santos EF, Silva AÂO, Leony LM, et al. Acute Chagas disease in Brazil from 2001 to 2018: A nationwide spatiotemporal analysis. PLoS Neglected Tropical Diseases. 2020;**14**(8):e0008445

[34] dos Santos VR, de Meis J, Savino W, et al. Acute phase of Chagas' disease in the Brazilian Amazon region: Study of 233 cases from Pará, Amapá and Maranhão observed between 1988 and 2005. Memorias do Instituto Oswaldo Cruz. 2018;**5**:e170298

[35] Díaz ML, Leal S, Mantilla JC, et al. Acute Chagas' outbreaks: Molecular and biological features of *Trypanosoma cruzi* isolates, and clinical aspects of acute cases in Santander, Colombia. Parasites & Vectors. 2015;**8**:1-14

[36] Maguire BJ, Dahal P, Rashan S, et al. The Chagas' disease study landscape: A systematic review of clinical and observational antiparasitic treatment studies to assess the potential for establishing an individual participant-level data platform. PLOS Neglected Tropical Diseases. 2021;**15**(8):e0009697608

[37] Messenger LA, Miles MA, Bern C. Between a bug and a hard place: Trypanosoma cruzi genetic diversity and the clinical outcomes of Chagas' disease. Expert Review of Anti-Infective Therapy. 2015;**13**(8):995-1029

[38] de Meis J, Morrot A, Farias-de-Oliveira DA, et al. Differential regional immune response in Chagas' disease. PLOS Neglected Tropical Diseases. 2009;**3**(7):e417

[39] Zhang L, Tarleton RL. Parasite persistence correlates with disease severity and localization in chronic Chagas' disease. The Journal of Infectious Diseases. 1999;**180**(2):480-486. DOI: 10.1086/314889

[40] Bonney KM, Luthringer DJ, Kim SA, et al. Pathology and pathogenesis of Chagas' heart disease. Annual Review of Pathology. 2018;**14**:421-447. DOI: 10.1146/annurev-pathol-020117-043711

[41] Ed S, Silva DKC, dos Reis BP, et al. Immunomodulation for the treatment of chronic chagas disease cardiomyopathy: A new approach to an old enemy. Frontiers in Cellular and Infection Microbiology. 2021;**11**:765879. DOI: 10.3389/fcimb.2021.765879

[42] Sabino EC, Ribeiro AL, Salemi V, et al. Ten-year incidence of Chagas' cardiomyopathy among asymptomatic *Trypanosoma cruzi*–seropositive former blood donors. Circulation. 2013;**127**(10):1105-1115

[43] Hasslocher-Moreno A, Xavier S, Saraiva R, et al. Progression rate from the indeterminate form to the cardiac form in patients with chronic Chagas' disease: Twenty-two-year follow-up in a Brazilian urban cohort. Tropical Medicine and Infectious Disease. 2020;**5**(2):76

[44] Viotti R, Vigliano C, Lococo B, et al. Long-term cardiac outcomes of treating chronic Chagas' disease with Benznidazole versus No treatment.

A Nonrandomized Trial. Annals of Internal Medicine. 2006;**144**:724-734

[45] Riarte A, Prado N, De Rissio AM et al. TRAENA: Benznidazole treatment in adult patients with low risk chronic Chagas' disease—A Phase 3 randomized clinical trial. Newsletter no. 6. plataforma de investigación clínica en enfermedad de Chagas' (Chagas' disease clinical research platform) 2016, Rio de Janeiro. p. 14. Available from: https://dndi.org/wp-content/uploads/2016/06/DNDi_Chagas'_Newsletter_6_ENGLISH_2016.pdf

[46] Morillo CA, Marin-Neto JA, Avezum A, et al. Randomized trial of benznidazole for chronic Chagas' cardiomyopathy. New England Journal of Medicine. 2015;**373**:1295-1306

[47] Rayner CR, Smith PF, Andes D. Model-informed drug development for anti-Infectives: State of the art and future. Clinical pharmacology & therapeutics. 2021;**109**(4):867-891

[48] Al Jalali V, Zeitlinger M. Systemic and target-site pharmacokinetics of antiparasitic agents, Clinical Pharmacokinetics. 2020;**59**:827-847

[49] Strauss M, Lo Presti MS, Ramírez JC, et al. Differential tissue distribution of discrete typing units after drug combination therapy in experimental Trypanosoma cruzi mixed infection. Parasitology. 2021;**148**:1595-1601

[50] Pérez-Mazliah D, Ward A, Lewis M. Host-parasite dynamics in Chagas' disease from systemic to hyper-local scales. Parasite Immunology. 2021;**43**:e12786

[51] Villar JC, Perez JG, Cortes OL, et al. Trypanocidal drugs for chronic asymptomatic Trypanosoma cruzi infection. Cochrane Database of Systematic Reviews. 2014;**5**:CD003463

[52] Chadalawada S, Sillau S, Archuleta S, et al. Risk of cardiomyopathy among patients with the acute phase or indeterminate form of Chagas' disease. A systematic review and Meta-analysis. JAMA Network Open. 2020;**3**(8):e2015072. DOI: 10.1001/jamanetworkopen.2020.15072

[53] Mendicino D. Rapid diagnostics test for detecting Chagas' disease—Breaking barriers to diagnosis access in remote areas. Clinical Microbiology and Infection. 2019;**4**:1-2

[54] Van Norman G. Decentralized clinical trials. The future of medical product development? JACC: Basic to Translational Science. 2021;**6**(4): 384-387

[55] Shen J, Swift B, Mamelok R, et al. Design and conduct considerations for first-in-human trials. Clinical and Translational Science. 2019;**12**:6-19. DOI: 10.1111/cts.12582

[56] WHO International Clinical Trials Registry Platform. Available from: https://trialsearch.who.int/Default.aspx

[57] US National Library of Medicine. Clinicaltrials.gov Trial Registry. Available from: https://clinicaltrials.gov/ct2/results?cond=Chagas+Disease&term=&cntry=&state=&city=&dist

[58] Saville BR, Scott M, Berry SM. Efficiencies of platform clinical trials: A vision of the future. Clinical Trials. 2016;**13**(3):358-366

[59] U.S. Department of Health and Human Services Food and Drug Administration. COVID-19: Master Protocols Evaluating Drugs and Biological Products for Treatment or Prevention Guidance for Industry. 2021. Available from: https://www.fda.gov/media/148739/download

[60] Rial MS, Seremeta KP, Esteva MI, et al. In vitro studies and preclinical evaluation of benznidazole microparticles in the acute *Trypanosoma cruzi* murine model. Parasitology. 2021;**148**(5):566-575

[61] Saraiva RM, Portela LF, GPE S, et al. Disulfiram repurposing in the combined chemotherapy of Chagas disease A protocol for phase I/II clinical trial. Medicine Case Reports and Study Protocols. 2021;**2**(7):e0110

[62] González-Herrera F, Cramer A, Pimentel P, et al. Simvastatin attenuates endothelial activation through 15-epi-lipoxin A4 production in murine chronic Chagas cardiomyopathy. Antimicrob Agents Chemother;**61**:e02137-e02116. DOI: 10.1128/AAC.02137-16

[63] Cevey AC, Mirkin GA, Donato M, et al. Treatment with Fenofibrate plus a low dose of Benznidazole attenuates cardiac dysfunction in experimental Chagas disease. International Journal for Parasitology: Drugs and Drug Resistance. 2017;**7**(3):378-387

[64] Vera-Ku M, Meza-González G, Carlier Y, et al. Comparison of methodologies for detecting *Trypanosoma cruzi* parasites by microscopic observation of microhematocrit capillary tubes. Revista da Sociedade Brasileira de Medicina Tropical. 2019;**52**:e20180505. DOI: 10.1590/0037-8682-0505-2018

[65] Pinto Dias JC. Acute Chagas' disease. Mem. Inst. Oswaldo Cruz, Rio de Janeiro. Revista da Sociedade Brasileira de Medicina Tropical. 1984;**79**:85-91. DOI: 10.1590/S0074-02761984000500017

[66] Pinto AY, Valente SA, Valente VAC, et al. Acute phase of Chagas' disease in the Brazilian Amazon region: Study of 233 cases from Pará, Amapá and Maranhão observed between 1988 and 2005. Revista da Sociedade Brasileira de Medicina Tropical. 2008;**41**(6):602-614

[67] Pinazo JM, Thomas M, Bua J, et al. Biological markers for evaluating therapeutic efficacy in Chagas' disease, a systematic review. Expert Review of Anti-infective Therapy. 2014;**12**(4):479-496

[68] Sguassero Y, Cuesta CB, Roberts KN, et al. Course of chronic *Trypanosoma cruzi* infection after treatment based on parasitological and serological tests: A systematic review of follow-up studies. PLoS One. 2015;**10**(10):e0139363

[69] Hagström L, Marques AL, Nitz N, Hecht M. The use of qPCR in human Chagas' disease: A systematic review. Expert Review of Molecular Diagnostics. 2019;**19**(10):875-894

[70] Sulleiroa E, Muñoz-Calderon A, Schijman A. Role of nucleic acid amplification assays in monitoring treatment response in Chagas' disease: Usefulness in clinical trials. Acta Tropica. 2019;**199**:105120

[71] Alonso-Padilla J, Lopez MC, Esteva M, et al. Serological reactivity against T. cruzi-derived antigens: Evaluation of their suitability for the assessment of response to treatment in chronic Chagas' disease. Acta Tropica. 2021;**221**:105990

[72] U.S. Food and Drug Administration Center for Drug Evaluation and Research Application Number: 209570orig1s000 Benznidazole Clinical Microbiology/Virology Review(s). 2016. p. 95. Available from: https://www.accessdata.fda.gov/drugsatfda_docs/nda/2017/209570Orig1s000MicroR.pdf

[73] U.S. Food and Drug Administration Center for Drug Evaluation and Research Application Number: 209570orig1s000

Benznidazole Clinical Review. 2016. p. 219. Available from: https://www.accessdata.fda.gov/drgsatfda_docs/nda/2017/209570Orig1s000MedR.pdf

[74] U.S. Food and Drug Administration Center for Drug Evaluation and Research Application Number: 13464orig1s000 Multi-Discipline Review Summary Review Nifurtimox. 2019. p. 297. Available from: https://www.accessdata.fda.gov/drugsatfda_docs/nda/2020/213464Orig1s000MultidisciplineR.pdf

[75] Hidron AI, Gilman RH, Justiniano J, et al. Chagas cardiomyopathy in the context of the chronic disease transition. PLOS Neglected Tropical Diseases. 2010;**4**(5):e688. DOI: 10.1371/journal.pntd.0000688

[76] Baldoni N, Quintino N, Alves G, et al. Quality of life in patients with Chagas' disease and the instrument used: An integrative review. Revista do Instituto de Medicina Tropical de São Paulo. 2021;**63**:e46. DOI: 10.1590/S1678-9946202163046

[77] Quintino ND, Sabino EC, da Silva JL, et al. Factors associated with quality of life in patients with Chagas' disease: SaMi-trop project. PLoS Neglected Tropical Diseases. 2020;**14**(5):e0008144

[78] The Voice of the Patient. A series of reports from the U.S. Food and Drug Administration's (FDA's)Patient-Focused Drug Development Initiative. Chagas' Disease. Report Date: November 2015. p. 20. Available from: https://www.fda.gov/media/94403/download

[79] Berman J, Radhakrishna T. The tropical disease priority review voucher: A game-changer for tropical disease products. The American Journal of Tropical Medicine and Hygiene. 2017;**96**(1):11-13. DOI: 10.4269/ajtmh.16-0099

[80] U.S. Department of Health and Human Services, Food and Drug Administration. Guidance for Industry Expedited Programs for Serious Conditions – Drugs and Biologics. 2014. Available from: https://www.fda.gov/media/86377/download

[81] European Medicines Agency. Orphan drug designation. Available from: https://www.ema.europa.eu/en/human-regulatory/overview/orphan-designation-overview. [Accessed: Dec, 2021]

[82] European Medicines Agency. Medicines for use outside the European Union. Available from: https://www.ema.europa.eu/en/human-regulatory/marketing-authorisation/medicines-use-outside-european-union. [Accessed: Dec, 2021]

[83] European Medicines Agency. PRIME-priority medicines. Available from: https://www.ema.europa.eu/en/human-regulatory/research-development/prime-priority-medicines. [Accessed: Dec, 2021]

[84] European Medicines Agency. Accelerated assessment. Available from: https://www.ema.europa.eu/en/human-regulatory/marketing-authorisation/accelerated-assessment. [Accessed: Dec, 2021]

Chapter 3

# The Saga of Selenium Treatment Investigation in Chagas Disease Cardiopathy: Translational Research in a Neglected Tropical Disease in Brazil

*Tania C. de Araujo-Jorge, Anna Cristina C. Carvalho, Roberto R. Ferreira, Luciana R. Garzoni, Beatriz M.S. Gonzaga, Marcelo T. Holanda, Gilberto M. Sperandio da Silva, Maria da Gloria Bonecini-Almeida, Mauro F.F. Mediano, Roberto M. Saraiva and Alejandro M. Hasslocher-Moreno*

## Abstract

This chapter describes the steps from basic research to the definition of a putative public health recommendation in the clinical protocols and therapeutic guidelines for selenium (Se) supplementation for patients with Chagas disease. From 1998 to 2018, we conducted a translational research project to test the concept that chronic Chagas disease cardiopathy (CCC) severity could be associated with low levels of blood selenium (Se), and if oral Se supplementation could help to sustain the asymptomatic cardiac stage and reduce disease severity. Pre-clinical studies in mice and a clinical trial conducted in the early asymptomatic cardiac stage of CCC patients (B stage) were performed, identified as "Selenium Treatment of Chagasic Cardiopathy (STCC)" trial. The roadmap of the selenium project was/is a real saga, with important obstacles that tested team resilience and revealed Brazilian conditions of science development. We discuss the main possible mechanisms involved in the physiopathology of CCC and the lessons learned in this process. In this chapter, we also organized the timeline of the translational project and described the crucial moments of the journey, as well as the next steps driving the research teams and their international and health industry connections.

**Keywords:** neglected tropical diseases, myocardiopathy, *Trypanosoma cruzi*, selenium, pathogenesis, poverty, translational research, trace elements, clinical trial

## 1. Introduction

From 1998 to 2018, we conducted a translational research project to test the concept that chronic Chagas disease cardiopathy (CCC) severity could be associated with low levels of blood selenium (Se), and if supplementation with Se could help to sustain the asymptomatic cardiac stage and reduce disease severity. Pre-clinical studies in mice [1–3], clinical studies in affected people [4], and a clinical trial [5] with patients in the early stages of CCC were performed. Here we revisit and build the narrative of this process, from the very first ideas, through all the difficulties that we faced until the present days and the perspectives to introduce a new treatment for a neglected disease.

## 2. Research in context

Chagas disease (CD) is caused by infection with the protozoa *Trypanosoma cruzi* and affects 6–7 million people, leading to 12,000 deaths annually in more than 21 countries, mainly in Latin America, where Brazil, Bolivia, and Argentina are the most affected nations [6]. CD is considered by the WHO as a neglected tropical disease, due to several factors such as (i) the global disinterest of the pharmaceutical industry related to the low-profit perspective in the development of new drugs and vaccines for a vulnerable population that is affected by the CD; (ii) related to social determinants of the affected population, including poverty, malnutrition, poor housing/sanitation, and low education levels [7]. As a consequence of the low investment in drug development for CD, only first-generation drugs dated from the seventies are currently in use for trypanocidal treatment—benznidazole (BZN) and nifurtimox (Nif). Nevertheless, it is estimated that only 1% of the infected persons are etiologically treated, due to the second dimension of negligence that is related to the negligence of public health policies to identify, diagnose, treat, and monitor chronically affected CD people.

To enhance the visibility to the real dimension of CD, WHO instituted a *World Chagas disease Day* in 2020 (https://www.who.int/campaigns/world-chagas-disease-day). The real dimension of CD worldwide is still only estimated, based on data that is more than 10 years old. In Brazil, national guidelines for therapeutics and clinical protocols (PCDT-Chagas) were adopted only in 2018 [8]. Treatment is recommended to prevent or reduce CD progression in both the acute and early chronic phases by using BZN or Nif [6]. About 20–30% of the infected persons will develop chronic complications related to cardiovascular and digestive systems, and CCC is the most relevant infectious heart condition in Latin America [6, 9, 10]. We recently reviewed the complex physiopathology of CCC and the possible interactions where Se could act to reduce oxidative damage that is caused by multiple determinants [11, 12]. **Figure 1** shows the main strategies that we could mobilize to face the complex physiopathogenesis of CD, which involves anti-parasite drugs (AP), modulators of inflammation (MI), immune stimulators (IS), regulators of pathology (RP), and the combination of different therapeutic strategies (CT).

The idea of using Se as a complementary treatment rises from its role in 25 human selenoproteins, some of them acting as antioxidants and others in endocrine and immune pathways [13, 14]. Therefore, the effect of Se therapy in CD development needed proof of concept related to experimental infection and in patients. Our group and other researchers are adding evidence in this direction.

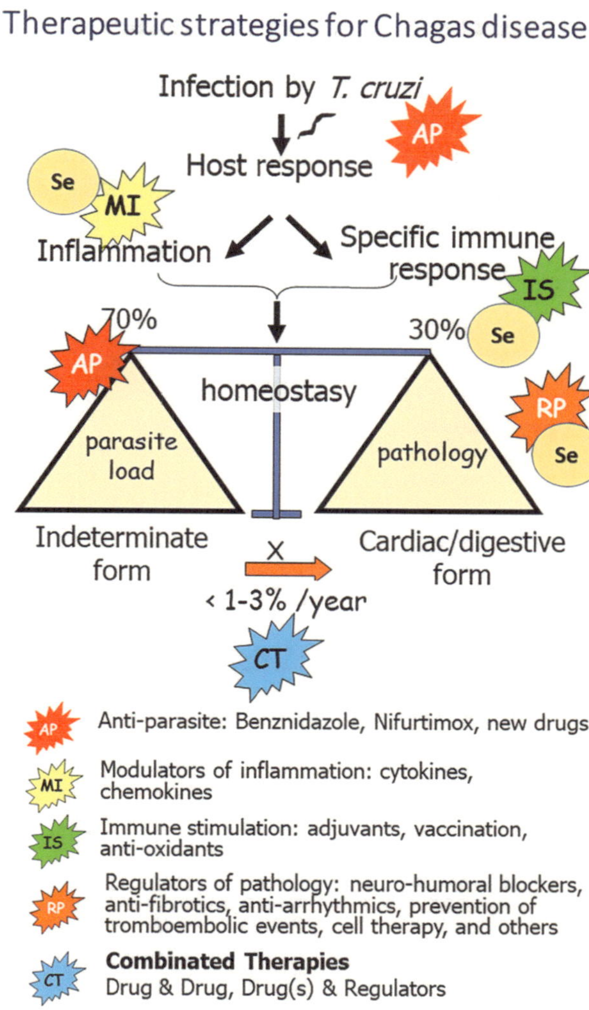


**Figure 1.**
*Five different therapeutic strategies that may be applied for Chagas disease treatment in the complexity of its multifactorial causality. Anti-parasite (AP) drugs such as benznidazole and nifurtimox, as well as others that are currently been studied, may reduce the parasite load in the early acute phase and in chronic infection when the parasite still evading the immune system. Infection in the hosts/patients triggers both local and systemic inflammation and a strong specific immune response. An adequate balance of these two mechanisms regulates the control of parasite growth and the regulation of physiopathology. Different strategies are under study in basic research for intervention in these four arms—Modulators of inflammation (MI), as cytokines, chemokines and their antagonists, immune stimulators (IS) as adjuvants, vaccines, and antioxidants, such as Se, regulators of pathology (RP) as neuro-humoral blockers, anti-fibrotic and anti-arrhythmic agents, prevention of thromboembolic events, cell therapy and others. The combination of different therapeutic strategies (CT) should help to face this complexity. However, the translation from basic to clinical studies and to patient access is still far.*

However, combined therapies are scarcely being tested in basic science [15, 16], and its translation to humans must also be investigated, mainly related to more clinical trials, as we performed for Se [5], opening more new doors than solving questions. As shown in **Figure 1**, the strategies of using combined trypanocidal chemotherapy and other agents to mitigate inflammatory disbalance, in which cytokine networks assume pathological roles, as well as increased fibrinogenic and neurodegenerative mechanisms, became co-protagonists in CD physiopathology [9, 10, 17].

## 3. Good beers and good ideas: the selenium hypothesis

In 1996, we were introduced to Se effects in cardiopathies through contact with Belgian colleagues that worked with *Médicins sans Frontières* in China and who studied experimental CD with us during a postdoctoral stage [18]. Good Belgian beers composed the scene for this open and free discussion. These colleagues were testing the use of Se to improve the treatment of Kashin-Beck osteoarthropathy [19], and they

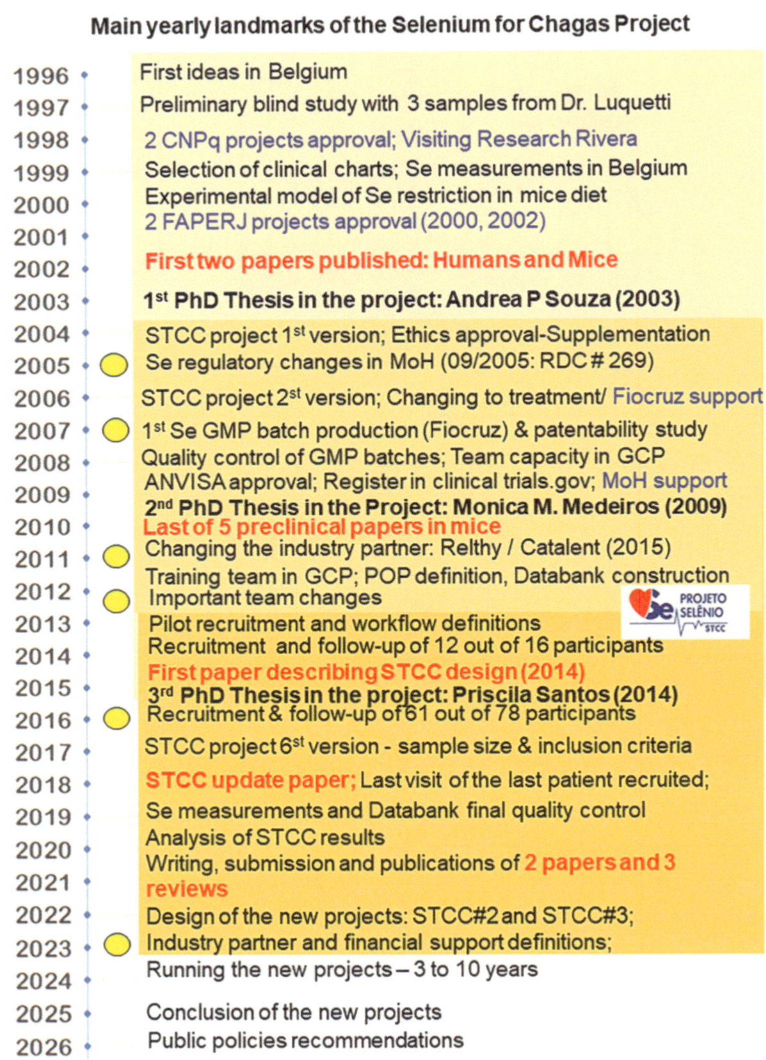


**Figure 2.**

*Main landmarks of the STCC clinical trial. Starting from the first ideas in 1996, three decades will lead to evidence to support public policies. Financial supports are shown in blue and main publications are shown in red; yellow dots at left indicate the critical points that threatened or delayed the project. The orange gradient background indicates the three main phases of the translational roadmap—(a) ideas, conceptualization, and basic preclinical studies, from 1996 to 2015, including the three PhD thesis, (b) pretrial activities conditioning the start of recruitment phase, from 2004 to 2014, and (c) the first clinical trial (STCC) from 2013 to 2020, with results published in 2021. This first trial used a short follow-up and showed a significant effect only in patients of the B2 stage of chronic Chagas cardiopathy, leaving some questions that implicated the design of new clinical trials to elucidate points that remained open, thus opening a fourth phase (white background) that deserves planning, financial funding, and implementation.*

were aware of Se involvement in an endemic cardiopathy, the Keshan disease [20]. Later, Keshan disease was linked to Se scarcity in the soil of some Chinese regions. Important projects were also conducted testing Se in an experimental virus disease and the possibility of pathology reversion after Se treatment [21]. Se deficiency in food turns benign viral strains into more virulent and pathogenic ones. The original idea was planted (a good idea)—does Se have any relationship with Chagas' disease cardiomyopathy?

We then asked Prof. Alejandro Luquetti, from the Federal University of Goiás, to give us some serum samples from CD patients at different stages of cardiac disease and measured Se levels. In the five pilot samples tested, two from non-infected and three from CD-infected people, we found that those with the lowest level of Se were the ones with the more advanced cardiac disease. It would be worth persisting in testing the hypothesis, thus starting the timeline of this long project. **Figure 2** shows this 30-year timeline, writing in black the yearly landmarks, in blue the application and approval of financial support projects, and in red the main publications.

## 4. Timeline of selenium treatment in Chagas Cardiopathy (STCC) clinical trial, the strength of a scientific network and the social arm of the project

The next step, in 1999, was to enhance the number of patients studied to confirm whether Se levels would be lower in patients with more severe cardiac disease. The first partnership was made with Dr. Alejandro M. Hasslocher-Moreno, who was the physician responsible for the clinic management and follow-up of CD patients at the Evandro Chagas National Institute of Infectious Diseases (INI), Fiocruz, Rio de Janeiro city. Se levels were measured and a very large variation was observed. We then decided that patients with different nutritional habits from another state in Brazil should also be analyzed. It implicated a new partnership with colleagues from Belo Horizonte city and CD patients from Dr. Manoel Otávio Rocha, enrolling a total of 273 patients in the study [4]. We observed that Se levels in patients with moderate and severe cardiopathy were lower than in patients with mild cardiopathy and indeterminate form, as well as in uninfected individuals [4].

In parallel, we performed some proof-of-concept studies, showing in experimentally *T. cruzi*-infected mice—(i) that Se diet deficiency turn mice much more susceptible to acute-phase mortality [1]; (ii) the parasite survival and replication was not affected by Se [2]; (ii) that mice parasitemia did not vary in situations of nutritional deficiency or Se supplementation [2]; (iii) that in the acute [2] and in the chronic [3] phases in mice, treatment with Se was able to reduce cardiac inflammation, regulate arrhythmias, and prevent cardiomegaly; (iv) digestive mega disease was prevented by Se supplementation [22]. A second idea was planted—could Se treatment or supplementation prevent the progression of chronic forms of CCC?

In 2004, we started to move on to the clinical trials stage. We designed a placebo-controlled, double-blind trial, recruiting patients with mild heart disease (stages B1 and B2 defined by the Brazilian Consensus on CD) followed at the Chagas clinic at INI-Fiocruz, for treatment of 100 mcg/day Se for 1 year. Two outcomes were defined—50% reduction in progression of heart disease and a significant reduction in left ventricular ejection fraction (LVEF) value in 5 years of follow-up. However, we did not previously contact a Se supplier. Our first impediment was to think that it should be easy to find a Se source in the Brazilian pharmaceutical market. The saga was in the early beginning. **Figure 2** represent the historical saga of the Se clinical trial, including the first step (1996–2004 period) of developing ideas, hypothesis, and pre-clinical studies.

1. In 2005, the Brazilian National Health Surveillance Agency (ANVISA), the drug regulatory agency, changed the criteria for daily supplementation dose of Se for 34.5 mcg. Therefore, the predicted dose of 100 mcg/day would be considered as treatment and not supplementation, implying the need to change the clinical trial regulatory licenses. Then, in June 2006, a second version of the trial was approved by the Ethics Committee.

2. In 2005, we found no Se supplier in Brazil under good manufacturing practices (GMP) conditions for clinical trials, either organic or inorganic. In sequence and based on the opportunity that Fiocruz has an industry sector for drugs and medicines production (FarManguinhos/Fiocruz), we tried a partnership for Se production, but it was not possible due to technical restrictions.

3. In 2006, the production was staggered at other Fiocruz industry sectors (Bio-Manguinhos/Fiocruz) and we initially succeeded. One year later we signed a contract and the first batch of liquid sodium selenite in ampoules was manufactured by BioManguinhos.

4. In June 2009, we submitted the essay proposal to ANVISA, which approved it in 5 months, after a single meeting for clarification and adjustments.

5. In early 2010, we received the bad news that BioManguinhos would have to interrupt the GMP production of Se due to a priority of the factory's response to the shortage of yellow fever vaccine.

6. We then started a journey to find a private industry partner. In 2011, based on the experience of the recently organized Fiocruz Clinical Research Platform (http://www.ppt.fiocruz.br/fiochagas/2021/09/27/quem-somos/), we found the *Relthy Co*., a national company as a partner that was interested in manufacturing Se and placebo under the same conditions. In 2011, a contract with *Relthy* was signed and we started the studies with the first batch of softgel capsules containing placebo or 100 mcg sodium selenite.

7. In 2013, the team that worked in the pre-clinical studies and that was initially trained for the clinical trial, was partially disarticulated with the departure of the project manager and other technicians.

8. In 2013, we reorganized the STCC team, with the completion of the database preparation and training of the new group in Good Clinical Research Practices (GCP). The database was structured with 389 fields to be filled in the Research Electronic Data Capture (REDCap), a web-based application to capture data for clinical research and create databases, divided into (i) Tracking and inclusion, (ii) Baseline visit for cardiac and clinical data (history and physical examination); (iii) Clinical follow-up, electrocardiogram (ECG) and echocardiogram (ECO); (iv) polymerase chain reaction for *T. cruzi*; (v) Se measurement; (vi) Thyroid hormones; (vii) Pregnancy test; (viii) Laboratory biomarkers; (ix) Clinical analyzes (hematology blood count and biochemistry);

(x) Immunological analyzes (humoral and cellular); (xi) Nutritional assessment; (xii) Follow-up ECG and ECO; (xiii) Follow-up echocardiogram. A challenge was the complexity of dealing with so many fields, multiplied by 135 expected participating patients multiplied by 14 visits each, with 10 only in the first year. It resulted in 1890 visits, with all the variables and biomarkers collected in most of them. In 2014, we had overcome the main obstacles to crossing the "valley of death," as shown in Declan Butler's publication in *Nature* in 2008 [23], and we the first patient was enrolled, enabling the publication of the STCC trial protocol in 2014 [24]. But then...

9. In 2015, the manufacturer *Relthy Co*. was purchased by a multinational company, Catalent, and we needed to re-discuss the clinical trial project Se supply and to renew the contract. Fortunately, the new partner agreed to maintain the project follow-up in 2015 and even prepared a second GMP batch.

10. On April 6th, 2016, a meeting of the external data safety monitoring board [24] was called to analyze some adverse effects recorded and to discuss the possible need for interrupting the clinical trial. Without the need of breaking the STCC blinding, this analysis concluded that a possibly intercurrent dengue virus endemic infection could have caused the noted effects (leukopenia/neutropenia) and the continuity of the trial was recommended. After ending the first year of STCC follow-up, the results published clearly confirmed the absence of adverse effects related to Se treatment [5].

11. During this long time, it occurred many advances in the knowledge about the effect of Se treatment in cancer and heart disease. It became clear that perhaps the dose provided in our clinical trial (100 mcg/day) could not be sufficient. From 2013 to 2018, four articles showed that 200 mcg was ideal for cardiovascular protection [25–28], and Swedish studies in elderly people proposed the benefits of the association of Se with the co-factor coenzyme Q10 for the expected outcomes. There was then a risk that STCC could end with no significant results, due to the lower concentration of Se chosen in 2004, based on cardiovascular literature related to Se treatment available at that time.

12. At the end of 2014, after 1 year of patients recruitment, we noted that the rate of recruitment was very slow (**Figure 3**), compromising the ability to reach the 163 volunteers needed for STCC protocol. It was 2015 when the third idea was planted—how to think about strategies to bring people with Chagas disease closer together and interest them in participating in the study to test/develop new medication and vaccines? Would it be possible to make them partners in the study or in actions to engage more patients in the knowledge of their own disease?

At this point, we decided to develop what we call the social arm of the clinical project.

April 14, 2015, we organized a meeting to make a public launch of the project, and to propose workshops of playful activities to "Talk about Chagas with Science and Art," inspired by the work of the Argentine group "Hablamos de Chagas" [29]. These initiatives quickly produced results—(i) we organized five successive editions of the course "We talk about Chagas with Science and Art" from 2015 to 2019, for people with CD, their family members, and health professionals; (ii) we created a

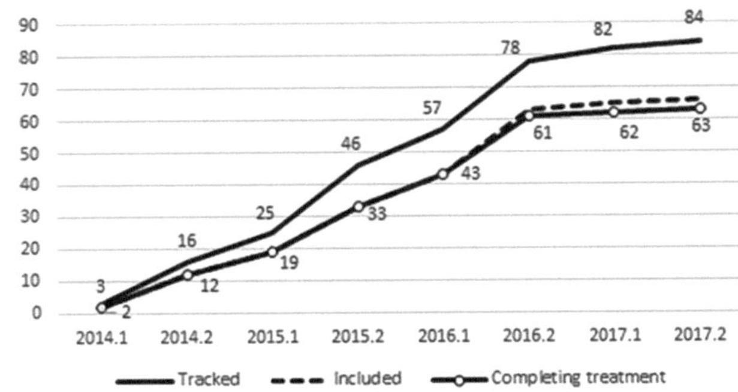


**Figure 3.**
*Time sequence of inclusion of participants on the STCC clinical trial. Black solid line shows the putative participants tracked, dashed line shows the participants included after signing the project voluntary consent form, and solid line with white dots shows the number of patients that completed the one-year treatment. Note that after 2015 the slope angle of the inclusion curve rise, denoting a success in the recruiting phase.*

"Rio Chagas Collective" on social media, which gave rise to the (iii) "Rio Chagas Association," founded on April 8, 2016, in which we participate in the Scientific Council; and (iv) the Rio Chagas Association participants inspired us to conceive the "Chagas Express XXI" social technology [30].

13. In 2018, we created a *YouTube* channel called "We talk about Chagas" (https://www.youtube.com/c/FalamosdeChagas) to provide videos about Chagas disease, and in 2019, we created the social technology for those affected by the disease named "Expresso Chagas XXI" to talk about Chagas in endemic areas, bringing science, culture, and art to those most in need of information for health promotion, prevention of Chagas disease and access to diagnosis and treatment in the Unified Health System (SUS – Sistema Único de Saúde). In 2019, we carried out a pilot expedition in four cities in an endemic area for CD in northern Minas Gerais. In addition, in 2020, we organized solidarity strategies for coping with the COVID-19 pandemic together with Rio Chagas Association (virtual WhatsApp meetings called "Coffee with Affection").

Chagas Express XXI was created as an "imaginary train" with around 40 ArtScience workshops, games, laboratory activities, and conversation circles. It was structured with an entry and exit point, followed by six more modules of activities that combined a focus on associations of affected people, on opportunities for the public to rediscover Carlos Chagas' discoveries, on microscopic observations and play, on health education in approach. A One Health approach was adopted, with a focus on home care, environment and reservoirs, and wellness activities. Chagas Express XXI was conceived as a social technology since all processes were co-created by scientists and patients with Chagas disease and worked with local cross-sector partnerships. We observed that 81% of the more than 2000 participants were unaware of the possibility of treating Chagas disease and 52% requested a blood test to diagnose CD. From the 1100 adults tested, 20% were diagnosed as positive for *T. cruzi* infection [30].

The fourth idea would then be: if the clinical trial of Se becomes unfeasible, we will have a social legacy to be able to continue later.

14. However, the problem was not only in the communication and mobilization of patients to participate in STCC, since in INI/Fiocruz cohort the number of patients

in the B1 and B2 stages of CCC was small as compared to patients in other clinical stages (indeterminate, A and C/D). Besides, a new risk for the project was arising: a long time had passed and the patients in the INI/Fiocruz cohort aged, acquiring comorbidities that were predicted as exclusion criteria and entering other studies that were ongoing, almost making the trial unfeasible due to a very slow rate of inclusion, as shown in **Figure 3**, during the years 2016 and 2017. To overcome this problem, the clinicians proposed to increase the age of recruitment from 65 to 75 years and to consider diabetes mellitus as a non-exclusion criterion.

Besides, the statisticians carried out other scenario studies for the feasibility of the STCC. They concluded that by extending the age range to up to 75 years, reducing the time of follow-up to one year, and focusing as a primary outcome only on the reduction of LVEF values (and not on the rate of CCC progression), we would conclude the inclusion of participants and generate some valid results. Then, in 2018, we published an update of the protocol [31] and started working to include 62 patients, divided into the two groups (placebo and Se treatment) for a follow-up of one year. We were then able to include all the expected patients and on August 8th, 2018, we were able to complete the last 12 months' visit of the last participant included.

15. The next step was to include all the laboratory and the nutritional data in the database, to run quality control for it, and to start the statistical analysis, both for descriptions of the clinical findings of participants and for comparisons between the placebo and Se-treated groups, as well as sub-group analyses, whenever possible. The study results were finally published in September 2021 [5]. When comparing the mean values of LVEF recorded in Se treated with the placebo group at baseline and after 1 year of follow-up, we did not find significant differences in the B1/B2 stages patients (overall), nor in the B1 stage patients, but found a significant effect ($p$ = 0.02) in the B2 stage patients (**Figure 4**).

After one year (**Figure 4**, gray bars), all the groups showed a lower mean of LVEF when compared to baseline values (**Figure 4**, black bars). However only those already on the B2 subgroup, with LVEF <45%, showed a high decrease in LVEF in 1-year, which

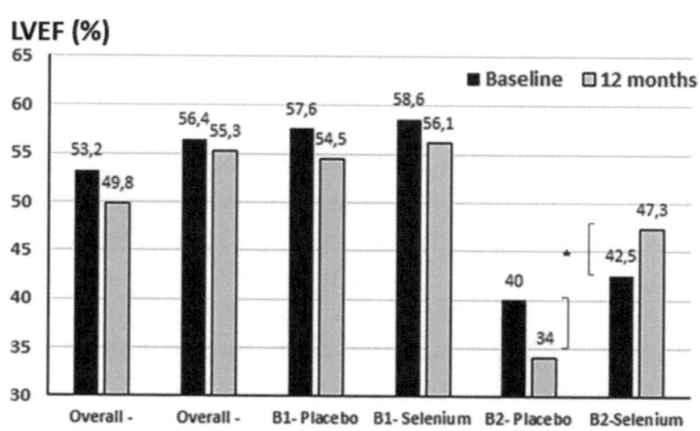


**Figure 4.**
*Mean values for left ventricular ejection fraction recorded for all the patients participating in the STCC clinical trial, at baseline (baseline, black bars) and after 12 months (gray bars). In the X-axis it is shown the comparison of the groups treated with placebo or selenium, considering all the participants in each group and in the subgroups B1 and B2 stages. For details, see reference #5.* ***Figure 4*** *Was prepared with data published in the STCC results [5].*

was reversed by Se treatment. The differences in LVEF longitudinal changes between groups were evaluated using linear mixed effect models in intention-to-treat analyses. This type of analysis assesses the rate of change of the outcomes by the time X intervention group interaction term, considering the correlations between repeated measures over time and missing data. In the B2 subgroup, the worsening of cardiac dysfunction was significantly reduced by Se treatment, and while the placebo group had a drop in LVEF, the Se group remained stable. In addition, only in the Se group, we observed cases of LVEF increase of more than 10 absolute points in 5 patients (n = 3) and recovery from stage B2 to B1 (n = 2), as reported [5]. In this short-term follow-up (1 year), the secondary outcomes observed were all related to LVEF as the underlying cause and could not be weighted in the analysis. We also observed that treatment with Se was safe for patients with CCC and that the low percentage of adverse effects detected were similar in the two groups. However, there was no complete shift of patients treated with Se to a safe range of serum Se (>100mcg/L), indicating that the dose of 100 mcg per day may have been insufficient. Further studies are needed to explore higher doses and/or associations of Se at different stages of CCC (B2 and C) at a short follow-up (one year) and at early diseases stages (A and B1), with longer follow-up.

16. The paper with STCC results [5] discussed some possibilities and pointed that "new clinical trials with a longer follow-up are needed to investigate the effects of Se in the mild (stages A and B) or severe (stages C and D) CCC, and in the asymptomatic indeterminate clinical form". The limitations of STCC were reported and the future outspread of the project is depicted in **Figure 2** from 2022 to, at least, 2026. The design of new projects (STCC#2 and STCC#3) is underway, and when the adequate industry partnership(s) will be signed, the proposal is that the new clinical trials will have a following of 3 to 10 years to generate the necessary evidence to support public policies recommendations.

## 5. Team resilience to face all the difficulties

From basic research to a putative public health recommendation in clinical protocols and therapeutic guidelines, the roadmap of the Se project was a real saga, with many obstacles that tested team resilience and Brazilian conditions of science development.

This resilience derived from the strength of the encounter between a basic research group (in Oswaldo Cruz Institute (IOC), founded by TCAJ) and a clinic research group (INI, founded by AMHM). Both groups were very active in producing new knowledge in CD and were excited with the idea of conceiving and performing the first Brazilian clinical trial [23] with a strategy based on one of the pathological mechanisms implicated in CCC [8, 9]. Overpassing all the difficulties that were listed in **Figure 2** (item 3), one after another, and attaining the conclusion of the trial gave even more strength to this partnership, our self-confidence, and our mutual respect increased.

The progress attained in the social arm of the project was also a source of resilience. More IOC/Fiocruz laboratories are associated with the project, as we could see from the Chagas Express publication [30] in August 2021. A project recently approved is preparing a virtual version of Chagas Express (https://expressochagas.com/), integrating contents related to COVID-19 as well as new expeditions to other endemic regions, planned for 2022.

In addition, this social arm of the project was developed at a very important moment in the struggle for the rights of patients with Chagas' disease. In 2018, the Ministry of Health, through its National Commission of Technology Incorporation, offered Therapeutic Guideline for CD Diagnosis and Treatment (PCDT Chagas) to public consultation, fostering discussions that lead to reformulations and publication in 2019. It was one of the main documents disseminated in the expedition to Minas Gerais by Expresso Chagas XXI [30]. We also participated in the advocacy movement that led to compulsory notification of chronic cases. Together with the traditional surveillance of cases in the acute phase, ordinance No. 1.061, May 18, 2020, introduced notification of chronic cases in Brazilian territory, strengthening the construction of public policies based on scientific evidence.

In a recent review [32], Morel discussed that CD is an example of successful translational research integrating basic and applied science, attaining the control of its transmission by insect vectors in large regions of the Southern Cone countries in the 90s. However, if the successful control of CD transmission by insect vectors is, in fact, a paradigmatic achievement in science translation, in addition to organizing a strong scientific community in Brazil and in Latin America, the translational research to focus on vaccines and treatments suffers extremely negative pressures as the ones we reported above. One important lesson to take home after this saga is that translational science on a neglected disease in *Innovative Developing Country, such* as Brazil, is not simple and needs specific policies to help scientists to overcome the valley of death. Morel also recognized that success in translation derives from "a long process led by incredible people, each one a leader in her or his area of work, who were able to collaborate with equally dedicated partners at the decision-making and political levels." As Morel reminded, thought the words of Lewis Carroll in his book, "Alice through the looking glass": "now, here, you see, it takes all the running you can do, to keep in the same place. If you want to get somewhere else, you must run at least twice as fast as that!"

## 6. Conclusions

What are the lessons learned and the next steps?

Four lessons were learned during the STCC saga—#1: the harmonious interaction between the clinical and basic research teams is essential to allow translational research to proceed; # 2: even in the pre-clinical phase, it is essential to identify potential suppliers in the market for the formulations that are intended to be used as treatment and/or industry partners interested in leading the product to the market; #3: the inclusion of master's and doctoral students should only be done in pre-clinical studies. In clinical trials, the stable inclusion of trained and mature professionals, economically stable, is necessary to avoid the shortage of human resources during the study; #4: a national and international network of experts is critical to overcoming the numerous doubts that arise in such a long study. In this case, we learned a lot about the clinical use of Se during the 15 years of the clinical trial, and we continue to learn about the physiopathology and clinical management of patients with Chagas disease.

Concerning the next steps, we are at the stage of preparing the reports for the sponsors and for our patients participating in the study. We will have several consequences in the clinical scope:

i. to carry out the cardiological follow-up of the study participants for another 4 to 10 years;

ii. to conduct a clinical trial with Brazil nuts as a natural source of Se;

iii. to identify PCR-*T. cruzi* positive patients at the end of the trial to treat them with benznidazole for 6 months plus Se;

iv. to accomplish the study of immunological biomarkers and gene polymorphism for cytokines and selenoproteins in samples from participants in the published study;

v. to contact suppliers and industry partners to enable further studies with Se in different settings, conditions, and associations and in multicenter and international arrangements.

As a second initiative, we will prepare a dossier for the National Commission of Technology Incorporation in the Health System (Comissão Nacional de Incorporação de Tecnologias no SUS" – CONITEC) to evaluate the recommendation of dietary supplementation for patients with Chagas disease with Se, either by supplementation with one Brazil nut per day (about R $20 per month) or by supplementation with Se and Coenzyme Q10 (about R$80 per month), due to type B levels of evidence for therapeutic studies in the literature and the safety when administering Se to elderly persons [25–27].

Last, but not least, we intend to incorporate Chagas Express XXI as cutting-edge educational technology, since we have already demonstrated its potential as an instrument of field epidemiology. In the next expeditions planned for 2022 in the states of Pernambuco, Goiás, and Minas Gerais, we will include a rapid test for a local screening of positive people and inclusion in the National Health System for diagnostic confirmation and clinical follow-up. We will also include a local digital electrocardiogram to screen for possible abnormalities related to Chagas disease in individuals with mild cardiac form/stage A. The Chagas Express XXI is a potentially useful social technology for health and science education and active search for chronic cases of disease of asymptomatic CD patients, contributing to the notification of chronic cases and their inclusion in the lines of care of PCDT-Chagas. Furthermore, this technology can be adapted to understand and cooperate in other potentially epidemic situations, especially related to other neglected diseases, such as leishmaniasis, tuberculosis, and arboviruses.

## Acknowledgements

We dedicate this work to all the patients who participate in the STCC trial, some of them contributing to the creation of the Rio Chagas Association. We thank all the basic and the clinical groups´ members of the Selenium project: Maria Teresa Rivera, Jean Vanderpas, Andrea P. Souza, Bianca P. Olivieri, Solange L. de Castro, Gabriel M. Oliveira, and Andrea P. Souza. Constança Britto, Otacílio C. Moreira, Erica R. Maciel, Fernanda M. Carneiro, Sérgio S. Xavier, Priscila F. Santos, Henrique H. Veloso, Pedro E.A.A. Brasil, Andrea S. de Sousa, Paula S. da Silva and Luiz Henrique C. Sangenis. We also thank Catalent Brasil Ltda for supplying free-of-charge sodium selenite and placebo for the STCC study. T.C.A-J represents Fiocruz in the Ibero-American New Tools for the Diagnosis and Evaluation of CD (NHEPACHA) network. This work was supported by the Department of the Industrial Complex and Innovation in Health from the Brazilian Health Ministry (IOC Fiotec IOC-001-LIV-11-2-1; 25380.001603/2017-2089), the governmental agencies CNPq (306184/2010-9, 309545/2014-5;313011/2018-4), FAPERJ (E26/151.506/99; Protocol 33); and the Innovation and the Research Vice-Presidencies of Fiocruz. Students who participated in the project received fellowships from Coordenação de Aperfeiçoamento de Pessoal do Ensino Superior (CAPES) related to their respective Fiocruz post-graduation courses.

## Conflict of interest

The authors declare no conflict of interest. The funders had no role in the design of the study nor in the writing of the manuscript, or in the decision to publish the results.

## Author details

Tania C. de Araujo-Jorge[1*], Anna Cristina C. Carvalho[1], Roberto R. Ferreira[1], Luciana R. Garzoni[1], Beatriz M.S. Gonzaga[1], Marcelo T. Holanda[2], Gilberto M. Sperandio da Silva[2], Maria da Gloria Bonecini-Almeida[3], Mauro F.F. Mediano[2], Roberto M. Saraiva[2] and Alejandro M. Hasslocher-Moreno[2]

1 Laboratory of Innovations in Therapies, Education and Bioproducts, Oswaldo Cruz Institute (IOC), Rio de Janeiro, RJ, Brazil

2 Laboratory of Clinical Research in Chagas Disease, Evandro Chagas National Institute of Infectious Diseases (INI) at Oswaldo Cruz Foundation (Fiocruz), Rio de Janeiro, RJ, Brazil

3 Laboratory of Immunology and Immunogenetic, Evandro Chagas National Institute of Infectious Diseases (INI) at Oswaldo Cruz Foundation (Fiocruz), Rio de Janeiro, RJ, Brazil

*Address all correspondence to: taniaaj@ioc.fiocruz.br

## References

[1] Souza AP, Oliveira GM, Nève J, Vanderpas J, Pirmez C, De Castro SL, et al. *Trypanosoma cruzi*: Host selenium deficiency leads to higher mortality but similar parasitemia in mice. Experimental Parasitology. 2002;**101**:193. DOI: 10.1016/s0014-4894(02)00134-0

[2] Souza AP, Oliveira GM, Vanderpas J, De Castro SL, Rivera MT, Araújo-Jorge TC. Selenium supplementation at low doses contributes to the decrease in heart damage in experimental *Trypanosoma cruzi* infection. Parasitology Research. 2003;**91**:51-54. DOI: 10.1007/s00436-003-0867-9

[3] Souza AP, Jelicks LA, Tanowitz HB, Olivieri BP, Medeiros MM, Oliveira GM, et al. The benefits of using selenium in the treatment of Chagas disease: Prevention of right ventricle chamber dilatation and reversion of *Trypanosoma cruzi*-induced acute and chronic cardiomyopathy in mice. Memórias do Instituto Oswaldo Cruz. 2010;**105**:746. DOI: 10.1590/S0074-02762010000600003

[4] Rivera MT, Souza AP, Hasslocher-Moreno A, Xavier SS, Gomes JAS, Rocha MOC, et al. Progressive Chagas' cardiomyopathy is associated with low selenium levels. The American Journal of Tropical Medicine and Hygiene. 2002;**66**:706. DOI: 10.4269/ajtmh.2002.66.706

[5] Holanda MT, Mediano MFF, Hasslocher-Moreno AM, Gonzaga BMS, Carvalho ACC, Ferreira RR, et al. Effects of selenium treatment on cardiac function in Chagas heart disease: Results from the STCC randomized trial. EClinicalMedicine. 2021;**40**:101105. DOI: 10.1016/j.eclinm.2021.101105

[6] WHO, World Health Organization. Chagas disease (American trypanosomiasis) [Online]. 2021. Available from: https://www.who.int/health-topics/chagas-disease# [Accessed: March 12, 2021]

[7] Briceño-León R, Galván JM. The social determinants of Chagas disease and the transformations of Latin America. Memórias do Instituto Oswaldo Cruz. 2007;**102**(suppl. 1):109-112. DOI: 10.1590/S0074-02762007005000095

[8] Brasil, Ministério da Saúde. Protocolo Clínico e Diretrizes Terapêuticas Doença de Chagas. Relatório N° 397. Out/2018. Available from: http://conitec.gov.br/images/Protocolos/Relatorio_PCDT_Doenca_de_Chagas.pdf

[9] Rassi A Jr, Marin-Neto JA, Rassi A. Chronic Chagas cardiomyopathy: A review of the main pathogenic mechanisms and the efficacy of aetiological treatment following the BENznidazole evaluation for interrupting Trypanosomiasis (BENEFIT) trial. Memórias do Instituto Oswaldo Cruz. 2017;**112**:224-235. DOI: 10.1590/0074-02760160334

[10] Velasco A, Morillo CA. Chagas heart disease: A contemporary review. Journal of Nuclear Cardiology. 2018;**27**:445-451. DOI: 10.1007/s12350-018-1361-1

[11] Araujo-Jorge TC, Rivera MT, Vanderpas J, Garzoni LR, Carvalho ACC, Waghabi MC, et al. Selenium, TGF-beta and infectious cardiopathy: Lessons from studies on host infection with *Trypanosoma cruzi*, the human Chagas disease. Biomolecules. 2022;**12**(3):349. DOI: 10.3390/biom12030349

[12] Araujo-Jorge TC, Ferreira RR. Translational research in Chagas disease: Perspectives in nutritional therapy

emerging from selenium supplementation studies as a complementary treatment. Mem Inst Oswaldo Cruz. 2022;**117**: e220001, 1-4

[13] Zakeri N, Kelishadi MR, Asbaghi O, Naeini F, Afsharfar M, Mirzadeh E, et al. Selenium supplementation and oxidative stress: A review. PharmaNutrition. 2021;**17**:1201. DOI: 10.1016/j.phanu.2021.100263

[14] Hasani M, Djalalinia S, Khazdooz M, Asayesh H, Zarei M, Gorabi AM, et al. Effect of selenium supplementation on antioxidant markers: A systematic review and meta-analysis of randomized controlled trials. Hormones. 2019;**18**:451-462. DOI: 10.1007/s42000-019-00143-3

[15] Vilar-Pereira G, Resende Pereira I, de Souza Ruivo LA, Cruz Moreira O, da Silva AA, Britto C, et al. Combination chemotherapy with suboptimal doses of Benznidazole and Pentoxifylline sustains partial reversion of experimental Chagas' heart disease. Antimicrobial Agents and Chemotherapy. 2016;**60**:4297-4309. DOI: 10.1128/AAC.02123-15.2016

[16] Vilar-Pereira G, Carneiro VC, Mata-Santos H, Vicentino AR, Ramos IP, Giarola NL, et al. Resveratrol reverses functional Chagas heart disease in mice. PLoS Pathogens. 2016;**12**(10):e1005947. DOI: 10.1371/journal.ppat.1005947

[17] Cristovão-Silva AC, Brelaz-de-Castro MC, Hernandes MZ, Pereira VRA. Chagas disease: Immunology of the disease at a glance. Cytokine & Growth Factor Reviews. 2021; **S135906101**(21):00073-00073. DOI: 10.1016/j.cytogfr.2021.10.001

[18] Araujo-Jorge T, Rivera MT, el Bouhdidi A, Daëron M, Carlier Y. An Fc gamma RII-, Fc gamma RIII-specific monoclonal antibody (2.4G2) decreases acute Trypanosoma cruzi infection in mice. Infection and Immunity. 1993 Nov;**61**(11):4925-4928. DOI: 10.1128/iai.61.11.4925-4928.1993

[19] Moreno-Reyes R, Suetens C, Mathieu F, Begaux F, Zhu D, Rivera MT, et al. Kashin-Beck osteoarthropathy in rural Tibet in relation to selenium and iodine status. The New England Journal of Medicine. 1998;**339**:1112-1120. DOI: 10.1056/NEJM199810153391604

[20] Loscalzo J. Keshan disease, selenium deficiency, and the Selenoproteome. The New England Journal of Medicine. 2014;**370**:1756-1760. DOI: 10.1056/NEJMcibr1402199

[21] Beck MA, Handy J, Levander OA. Host nutritional status: The neglected virulence factor. Trends in Microbiology. 2004;**12**(9):417-423. DOI: 10.1016/j.tim.2004.07.007

[22] Souza AP, Sieberg R, LI H, Cahill HR, Zhao D, Araujo-Jorge TC, Tanowitz HB, Jelicks LA. The role of selenium in intestinal motility, morphology and inflammation in a murine model of Trypanosoma cruzi infection. Parasitology Research. 2010;**106**:1263-1267. DOI: 10.1007/s00436-010-1794-1

[23] Butler D. Translational research: Crossing the valley of death. Nature. 2008;**453**:840-842. DOI: 10.1038/453840a

[24] Brasil PEAA, Souza AP, Hasslocher-Moreno AM, Xavier SS, Passos SRL, Moreira MFR, et al. Selenium treatment and Chagasic Cardiopathy (STCC): Study protocol for a double-blind randomized controlled trial. Trials. 2014;**15**:388. DOI: 10.1186/1745-6215-15-388

[25] Alehagen U, Johansson P, Bjornstedt M, Rosen A, Dahlstrom U. Cardiovascular mortality and N-terminal-proBNP reduced after combined selenium and coenzyme

Q10 supplementation: A 5-year prospective randomized double-blind placebo-controlled trial among elderly Swedish citizens. International Journal of Cardiology. 2013;**167**:1860. DOI: 10.1016/j.ijcard.2012.04.156

[26] Alehagen U, Aaseth J, Johansson P. Reduced cardiovascular mortality 10 years after supplementation with selenium and coenzyme Q10 for four years: Followup results of a prospective randomized double-blind placebo-controlled trial in elderly citizens. PLoS One. 2015;**10**:e0141641. DOI: 10.1371/journal.pone.0141641

[27] Alehagen U, Alexander J, Aaseth J. Supplementation with selenium and coenzyme Q10 reduces cardiovascular mortality in elderly with low selenium status. A secondary analysis of a randomized clinical trial. PLoS One. 2016;**11**:e0157541. DOI: 10.1371/journal.pone.0157541

[28] Rayman MP, Wintherb KH, Pastor-Barriusoc R. Effect of long-term selenium supplementation on mortality: Results from a multiple-dose, randomized controlled trial. Free Radical Biology & Medicine. 2018;**127**:46. DOI: 10.1016/j.freeradbiomed.2018.02.015

[29] Sanmartino M, Mengascini A, Menegaz A, Mordeglia C, Ceccarelli S. Miradas Caleidoscópicas sobre el Chagas. Una experiencia educativa en el Museo de La Plata. Revista Eureka sobre Enseñanza y Divulgación de las Ciencias. 2012;**9**(2):265-273

[30] Araujo-Jorge TC, Ferreira RR, Rocha RMC, Vieira TM, Costa ND, Santos LL, et al. "Chagas express XXI": A new ArtScience social technology for health and science education—A case study in Brazilian endemic areas of Chagas disease with an active search of chronic cases. PLoS Neglected Tropical Diseases. 2021;**15**(7):e0009534. DOI: 10.1371/journal.pntd.0009534

[31] Holanda MT, Mediano MFF, Hasslocher-Moreno AM, Xavier SS, Saraiva RM, Sousa AS, et al. Protocol update for the selenium treatment and Chagasic cardiomyopathy (STCC) trial. Trials. 2018;**19**:507. DOI: 101186/s13063-018-2889-8

[32] Morel CM. Significance of a neglected tropical disease: Lessons from a paradigmatic case of 'success in translation'. Memórias do Instituto Oswaldo Cruz. 2021;**116**:e200277. DOI: 10.1590/0074-02760200277

Chapter 4

# Translational Research on Chagas Disease: Focusing on Drug Combination and Repositioning

*Marcos André Vannier-Santos, Ana Márcia Suarez-Fontes, Juliana Almeida-Silva, Alessandra Lifsitch Viçosa, Sandra Aurora Chavez Perez, Alejandro Marcel Hasslocher-Moreno, Gabriel Parreiras Estolano da Silveira, Luciana Fernandes Portela and Roberto Magalhães Saraiva*

## Abstract

Chagas disease, caused by the protozoan *Trypanosoma cruzi*, is a major neglected disease endemic to Latin America, associated to significant morbimortality comprising a remarkable socioeconomic problem mainly for low-income tropical populations. The present chapter focuses translational research on Chagas disease, approaching drug combinations and repositioning, particularly exploiting the parasite oxidative stress by prospecting prooxidant compounds combined with antagonists of antioxidant systems, for developing low-cost and safe therapies for this infection. The pertinent literature on protozoal parasitic diseases is reviewed as well as on repurposing disulfiram aiming the combination with the Chagas disease drug of choice benznidazole. Both disulfiram and its first derivative sodium diethyldithiocarbamate (DETC) are able not only to inhibit p-glycoprotein, possibly reverting resistance phenotypes, but also to reduce toxicity of numerous other drugs, heavy metals, etc. Therefore, this innovation, presently in clinical research, may furnish a novel therapeutic for *T. cruzi* infections overcoming the adverse effects and refractory cases that impair the effectiveness of Chagas disease treatment.

**Keywords:** drug combination, drug repositioning, translational medicine, Chagas disease, oxidative stress, *Trypanosoma cruzi*

## 1. Introduction

Chagas disease (CD), the parasitic infection caused by the kinetoplastid protozoan *Trypanosoma cruzi*, is also known as American trypanosomiasis, for the huge endemic areas in South and Central Americas [1], but autochthonous human [2–4] and domestic/wild animal [5–8] cases were reported in the United States, and due to migration, it is already considered a public health problem on a global scale reaching different continents [9–11]. It is noteworthy that climate changes may promote the northward insect vector propagation [12], possibly generating new foci or endemic areas, and suitable climatic conditions may be available in African and Asian nations [13]. Besides the vector bloodmeal, congenital, blood transfusion and organ transplantation [14], CD may be transmitted orally via food and beverages contaminated by triatomine feces such as sugarcane and açai juices [15, 16] and even water, stored in/near domiciles in arid regions [15, 16], as the parasite is able to survive in such media [17].

It is alarming that 6–7 million people are estimated to have CD worldwide, with *circa* 173,000 new cases/year and over 75 million people are at risk. CD is the parasitic disease of highest mortality in Latin America as 9490 deaths were reported in 2019. Furthermore, the real prevalence is largely unknown as most chronic patients are asymptomatic and even symptomatic patients have poor access to health public system. CD is endemic in 21 countries in Central and Latin America where about 5.7 million people have CD and 25% of the population is at risk [18]. In 2020, it was estimated that there were 3.2 million infected people, which can reach 1.5% of the general population. In addition, about 70 million are at risk of infection [19]. The prevalence of CD is presumably vastly underestimated. In January 2020, a study carried out by the ArtScience Initiative for Health Promotion, carried out by Oswaldo Cruz Foundation (Fiocruz) and collaborating organizations, showed a CD seropositivity of 20% in a tested population of an endemic area [20]. It must be mentioned this study was not designed to access CD prevalence and was biased by the population intention to get diagnosis procedures.

CD represents economic losses in excess of $1.2 billion/year to endemic countries in South America, in addition to more than $7 billion a year at global levels [21], including treatment and loss of productivity. Since no proven effective and approved vaccines are available for this disease, chemotherapy represents the only therapeutic intervention, as well as an important way to control them.

CD etiological treatment is directed according to the phase and clinical presentation of the disease, which is mandatory in the acute phase, congenital cases, or reactivation due to immunosuppression. In the chronic phase, the trypanocidal treatment is indicated in children and adolescents, recent infection, and women of childbearing age [22].

## 2. Therapeutics

Although CD was discovered and is studied for over a century [14], the etiologic treatment is still based on solely two drugs (**Figure 1**): the nitrofuran derivative nifurtimox (NFX; Lampit®, Bayer; 5-nitrofuran(3-methyl-4-(5′-nitrofurfurylideneamine) tetrahydro-4H-1,4-tiazine-1,1-dioxide), and the 2-nitromidazole benznidazole (BZ; LAFEPE; N-benzyl-2-nitroimidazole-acetamide) [23]. Both NFX and BZ were shown to produce remarkable ultrastructural alterations in mammal cells and tissues [24, 25], which were apparently more pronounced in NFX-treated animals [26]. Therefore, experimental chemotherapy studies approaching parasites as *T. cruzi* should preferentially include ultrastructural analysis, in order to offer a subcellular compartmentation understanding to aid the antiparasitic agent mechanism(s) of action elucidation [27, 28] and ultimately leading to the understanding of cell death pathways involved [29].

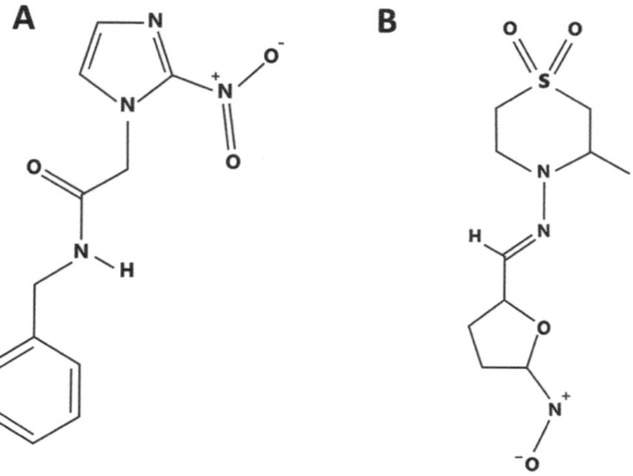


**Figure 1.**
*Molecular structures of the nitroheterocyclic drugs employed in the treatment of Chagas disease: the 2-nitroimidazole benznidazole (A) and the 5-nitrofuran nifurtimox (B).*

The CD therapeutics remain unsatisfactory, as they are associated with adverse effects [30–32], affecting 84.8 and 95.2% of patients treated with BZ and NFX, respectively [33], which may be severe, leading to the irreversible suspension of therapy in CD, in ≈20% [34, 35], ≈30% [36, 37], 41.5% [38], and up to 50% of the cases [39, 40]. Treatment suspension using NFX was reported in 43.8% of patients [33]. In an early study based on small samples, NFX was reported to be associated to definitive treatment interruption in 75% of patients [38]. Nevertheless, treatment intolerance was reported at similar levels with the use of the two drugs, approached by the same team [34, 35], but adverse effects, including neuropsychiatric events, may be more frequently associated to NFX [33]. In addition, it was reported that among patients who had discontinued BZ treatment and were treated with NFX, 12.3% also developed adverse effects that required definitive discontinuation of therapy [39]. Nevertheless, NFX was reported to be safe as a second-line therapy in patients who discontinued BZ [41].

Most CD patients are not treated because of the insufficient diagnosis and low cure rates observed in chronically infected patients [42], although treatment may diminish the disease progression and cardiovascular events [43, 44]. In addition, the CD treatment accomplishes only a parasitological cure, and a clinical cure is hardly proved [43, 45]. Whereas the *bona fide* sterile cure or complete clearance of the infection is considered a "prerequisite" for new anti-*T. cruzi* drug candidates [46], it is usually not achieved in murine model [47, 48] or human infection as immunosuppression often leads to infection reactivation [49]. In this regard, *T. cruzi* amastigotes may persist in a dormant or quiescent form, which may protect the parasites from antiparasitic agents [50, 51].

As the dormancy state of *T. cruzi* amastigotes is associated to drug resistance [50, 51], it is desirable to develop drugs able to affect dormant parasites. The mechanisms that allow the establishment of persistence include the capacity to suppress the oxidative burst produced by phagocytes largely depending on iron-containing superoxide dismutases (FeSOD) and trypanothione-acting enzymes [52]. Thus the use of disulfiram (DSF) is of potential relevance since it can diminish glutathione levels [53, 54], and the DETC first derivative of DSF is an SOD inhibitor [55, 56].

Furthermore, DSF could target *T. cruzi* dormancy. Although the signal transduction pathways involved in this process were not completely elucidated, it is interesting that DSF is able to reverse HIV latency affecting PKC (protein kinase C), AKT (protein kinase B), PI3K (phosphoinositide 3-kinases), NF-kB (nuclear factor kappa-light-chain-enhancer of activated B cells) [57, 58], which also affect *T. cruzi* infection [59, 60] that leads to the activation of PI3K [61], whereas DSF promotes PI3K inhibition [62].

An important study [63] approached the persistent parasite elimination, but the use of higher BZ doses might pose higher risks for patients. In this regard, the polyamine and thiol synthesis *Leishmania* are associated to macrophage M2 phenotype, leading to parasite persistence [64].

### 2.1 Drug resistance

Besides considerable severe adverse effects, one of the greatest problems of CD therapeutics is the selection of resistant parasites, impairing its effectivity, therefore causing refractory cases. BZ and NFX resistance is readily developed *in vitro* and *in vivo* [47, 65], in the former case, via different mechanisms that can act in concert [66].

Despite significant time and resources investments by innumerous research institutions over the world, only a few therapeutic candidates advanced the pipeline to treat neglected diseases such as CD [67]. It is alarming that it usually takes over 10 years to develop new drugs, whereas resistant parasites are rapidly selected. Also, there are naturally resistant *T. cruzi* strains [68–70] that express a novel ABCG-like transporter [71]. Besides extrusion pumps, *T. cruzi* resistance may involve SOD and trypanothione (*vide infra*). Therefore, there is pressing demand for the development of novel effective therapies for CD.

## 3. Oxidative stress in Chagas disease

Oxidative stress is a central phenomenon involved in aging, cancer, transmissible or infectious diseases, including COVID-19 [72], nontransmissible chronic conditions, such as metabolic diseases, autoimmune and degenerative disorders, inflammation, metal poisoning, etc. [73–75], produced by the imbalance on the production/uptake of oxidant/antioxidant species [76].

A plethora of antioxidant defenses evolved in order to balance the redox homeostasis [76, 77]. Oxidant species such as superoxide ($O_2^{\bullet-}$) and hydrogen peroxide ($H_2O_2$) are detoxified by SOD and catalase, respectively. Most cells rely also on the peptide glutathione (GSH), able to chelate reactive oxidant species (ROS) via cysteine sulfhydryl (SH) group and function as substrate for enzymes including GSH reductase and GSH peroxidase [78].

Although most of these processes are evolutionary conserved, some of the antioxidant defenses pathways differ between mammals and pathogens, therefore comprise potential chemotherapy targets. Contrary to mammals, GSH in trypanosomatid parasites mostly takes part in the adduct with the polyamine spermidine, forming *N*1,*N*8-bis(glutathionyl)spermidine (trypanothione, TSH), and therefore its expression depends on the GSH, TSH [79], and polyamine [80] metabolism pathways.

Metabolomics and gene expression studies [81] reveal the participation of both GSH and the spermidine synthesis pathway, indicating the participation of trypanothione, in the regulation of redox metabolism in trypanosomatids. GSH is very relevant not only in oxi-reductive homeostasis, as this molecule is also related to detoxification and resistance to different drugs/xenobiotics in tumor cells [82, 83] binding to drugs that are extruded via multidrug resistance transporters [84]. TSH binding to NFX and BZ is involved in the detoxication of these trypanocides [85, 86]. Therefore, glutathione/trypanothione can promote the action/reverse resistance to different drugs. *T. cruzi* parasites overexpressing trypanothione synthetase tolerated higher doses of BZ and NFX [87]. Conversely, the GSH biosynthesis inhibition using buthionine sulfoximine increases the efficacy of NFX and BZ upon *T. cruzi in vitro* [88] and NFX *in vivo* [89] as well as of stibogluconate on *Leishmania (L.) donovani* [90].

Interestingly, polyamine play pivotal roles in parasite cells [91, 92], including *T. cruzi* antioxidant defense [93], and its synthesis and transport pathways provide valuable chemotherapy targets [94, 95], including repositioned drugs [96].

Parasitic diseases such as CD are correlated to oxidative stress [97, 98], associated to triggered chronic inflammatory reactions [99, 100]. Endogenous oxidative stress may be produced by cell organelles, mainly mitochondria [101, 102]. The CD myocarditis is characterized by intense oxidative stress due both to inflammatory response associated to neutrophils and macrophages NADPH oxidase (Nox) activity and the macrophage superoxide produced by Nox2 is required for parasite control in early infection [103]. The mitochondrial ROS produced by cardiomyocytes plays a relevant role in intracellular oxidative stress and inflammation, causing myocardium tissue damage [104–106]. These events are not independent since mitochondrial ROS may trigger proinflammatory cytokines via NFkB and PARP/PAR pathways [107], and the mitochondrial MnSOD activity may revert much of the inflammatory foci and necrosis [105], and ineffective antioxidant defense is associated to oxidative stress [108]. Exosome or extracellular vesicles liberation may also contribute to inflammation and oxidative stress [107, 109]. The oxidative stress is also involved in neurodegeneration in both cardiac and gastrointestinal tissues [110]. The chronic oxidative stress in the nervous tissue is associated to cognitive deficit, which can be reversed by BZ treatment [111].

Thus, the use of adjuvant antioxidant agents may ameliorate the cardiac pathogenesis [107, 112, 113]. Interestingly, vitamin C, widely considered antioxidant, can at high concentrations also function as a prooxidant, undergoing pH-dependent autoxidation, leading to $H_2O_2$ formation [114, 115]. In CD models, ascorbic acid can also reduce parasitemia, promote BZ action, and enhance animal survival in murine infection [116, 117].

ROS production comprises a well-known microbicidal immune effector mechanism [118]; therefore parasite borne antioxidant systems are not only virulence factors [119]. Besides the parasiticidal activity, ROS may function as signaling molecules promoting parasite proliferation. As in the Paracelsus adage, "The dose makes the poison" (Latin: *sola dosis facit venenum*), ROS in mammalian cells may trigger different responses depending on concentration. Low ROS levels may have signal transduction roles, inducing responses such as activation, proliferation, and differentiation, whereas at higher levels such molecules are generally cytotoxic, leading to cell death [120]. Similarly, in *T. cruzi*, low ROS levels may signal for parasite invasion of host macrophages [121] and proliferation mainly in the acute phase [122], but high ROS levels culminate in programmed cell death, which may be inhibited by enhanced SOD expression [87]. Interestingly *T. cruzi* amastigotes undergo stress-induced proliferation [123].

## 4. Oxidative stress as a source of chemotherapy targets

Numerous therapeutic strategies exploit redox systems [124], including protozoal diseases [125], such as CD [126]. Therefore, antioxidant systems including SOD, trypanothione, and enzymes action on this glutathione-spermidine adduct (*N*1,*N*8-bis(glutathionyl)spermidine), such as trypanothione reductase, can comprise important chemotherapy targets [127]. Natural products such as the naphthoquinones α-/β-lapachones [128–130] and their derivatives [131, 132] have microbicidal activity against *T. cruzi*, among other pathogens [132]. Interestingly, β-lapachone derivatives were shown to cause mitochondrial dysfunction [131], damage [133], and autophagy, including mitophagy as well as apoptosis and necrosis [134]. In this regard, mitochondria comprise important therapeutical targets for cancer [135], aging [136], cardiovascular diseases [137], and degenerative diseases such as rheumatoid arthritis [138], Alzheimer's disease [139], Parkinson's disease [140], etc. Mitochondria are also promising target for antiparasitic [141, 142] and particularly antiprotozoal [143–145] therapeutic agents, specifically approached in trypanosomatids [146–148].

Up to 2% of the $O_2$ reaching the mitochondrial matrix is converted to $O_2^{\bullet-}$ (superoxide anions) forming $H_2O_2$ via SOD [149]. Like mammalian cells, *T. cruzi* mitochondria are a source of ROS [150] producing superoxide. Therefore, the Mn-SOD is important for controlling oxidative stress in this redox organelle. Contrary to mammals, the trypanosomatid mitochondria present FeSOD [151] that can protect from $O_2^{\bullet-}$ produced by macrophages [152].

Because of the prooxidant effects of antiparasitic drugs [126, 153–155], ROS detoxifying systems may comprise valuable scape mechanisms from pharmaceutical intervention [156] and programmed cell death triggered by mitochondrial $O_2^{\bullet-}$ [157].

The prooxidant capacity of both NFX and BZ, particularly in the former, is due to redox cycling with the production of $O_2^{\bullet-}$ [126, 158–160]. Superoxide may be not produced by BZ in the parasite, but in the host cell [161]. Therefore, FeSOD is linked to BZ resistance in *T. cruzi* [66, 162, 163]. Proteome of BZ-resistant *Trypanosoma cruzi* revealed enhanced FeSOD activity [164]. BZ resistance was associated to decreased cytosolic SOD but enhanced mitochondrial MnSOD and tryparedoxin-1 [165]. The deletion of the *sodb1* gene enhances *Trypanosoma brucei* susceptibility to BZ and NTX [166]. FeSOD is also implicated in drug resistance in *L.* (*Viannia*) *braziliensis* and *L.* (*Leishmania*) *infantum* [167, 168] *Entamoeba histolytica* [169]. Tryparedoxin peroxidase is also associated to antimony resistance in *L.* (*V.*) *braziliensis* [170]. In addition, SOD inhibition was reported to decrease parasitemia in *T. cruzi* murine infection [171].

Sirtuins are a highly conserved family of enzymes that deacetylate lysine residues on histone and non-histone proteins, using $NAD^+$ as a cosubstrate, regulating cellular antioxidant/Redox mechanisms [172, 173]. It is noteworthy that SIRT3, 4, and 5 are found in the mitochondrial matrix [174]. As cardiomyocyte mitochondrial dysfunction plays a central role in chagasic myocarditis (*vide supra*), the activation of sirtuins such as SIRT1 by agonists including resveratrol may enhance antioxidant defenses [175], and SIRT3 activates MnSOD, scavenging ROS [176]. Nevertheless, the sirtuin TcSir2rp3 was shown to increase *T. cruzi* resistance to BZ and NTX for overexpressing TcFeSOD-A activities [177].

Selenium and selenium-containing compounds show beneficial effects both in murine [178–180] and human *T. cruzi* infection [181, 182], therefore comprise

*DOI: http://dx.doi.org/10.5772/intechopen.104231*

promising coadjuvant therapies for CD [183–185], although selenium was previously reported to increase tissue parasitism [186].

This activity maybe largely dependent on redox regulation as this inflammatory infection is associated with intense oxidative stress, and selenium may be antioxidant [187] and anti-inflammatory [188], as well as catalyze hydrogen peroxide ($H_2O_2$) reduction [189], therefore possibly diminishing the oxidative stress in infected cardiomyocytes, by impairing the Fenton reaction in the presence of iron.

## 5. Repositioning and combining drugs

The combination of different drugs may pose the advantage of supra-additive effects, which may be synergistic, in parasite models such as *T. cruzi* [190], *Plasmodium falciparum*, *Trypanosoma rhodesiense* [191]. The identification of synergistic combinations is relevant since they tend to present higher selective indices [192, 193], consequently, avoiding side effects and potentially permitting development of antiparasitic agents used at lower concentrations.

The identification of drug combinations with multiple targets can lead to the use of novel multitarget mechanisms able to cope with the challenge of multigenic diseases [194] and/or chronic infections with complex pathophysiology. It is noteworthy that the pharmaceutical properties of the combination may be absent in the components alone [195], generating the innovative concept or science field termed polypharmacology with numerous applications on drug repurposing [196] and CD [197]. As the philosopher Aristotle (384–322 B.C.) stated: "The whole is greater than the sum of its parts."[1]

Furthermore, drug combinations are largely employed for preventing drug resistance [198–204]. However, this strategy is not constantly successful as the reports of resistance to the sulfadoxine-pyrimethamine combination began in the same year this antimalarial regimen entered the clinic [205]. Similarly, the discovery of artemisinin (ART) costed Youyou Tu over 30 years of hard work [206] and was worthy a Nobel Prize, but *P. falciparum* resistance to the drug was detected after about 10 years of use [207]. The antimalarial combination therapies based on the use of ART were considered key to the elimination of malaria [208], but in the very same year [209, 210] and even earlier [211], the arteminisin derivatives combination therapy failures were reported. In the case of CD, the problem may be even more upsetting as natural resistance isolates are arising, particularly in the Amazon region (*vide supra*). Thus, effective strategies to prevent different mechanisms of drug resistance to arise are immediately needed.

Approaching repositioned drugs with available pharmacokinetic and toxicological properties can shorten the long and expensive path between *in vitro* trials and new drugs. While the period between drug discovery and approval can be 12–16 years at a cost of US$1–2 billion, repositioned drugs can enter the clinic in ½ the time, at *circa* 1/3 the cost [212], with much higher success rates [213].

Drug repositioning maybe a promising approach in CD [214–227]. Similarly, drug combinations may be instrumental in CD [197, 228–233], and both strategies may be employed and associated [214, 234–236]. Furthermore, drug combinations can

[1] "Since that which is compounded out of something so that the whole is one, not like a heap (...), then, is something-not only its elements (...) but also something else (...)" 'Metaphysics' Book VII by Aristotle, Translated by W. D. Ross, often misquoted or mistranslated.

increase success of drug repositioning [237]. In addition, it was accurately hypothesized that the combined use of repurposed drugs with BZ could be more efficacious than BZ alone [238].

### 5.1 Repositioning disulfiram

Disulfiram (DS, 1,1′-disulfanediylbis(N,N-diethylmethanethioamide) also termed tetraethylthiuram disulfide; CAS no. 97-77-8; Molecular Formula: $C_{10}H_{20}N_2S_4$), a repositioned drug used in alcoholism and marketed as Antabuse® (**Figure 2**), was approved for medical use over 70 years ago and is widely used since then [239, 240].

At the very beginning, the discovery of thiocarbamates and its derivatives was serendipitous and showed clear signs of versatile perspectives that unequivocally culminated in the present promising repurposing strategies for both pharmaceutical and industrial applications [241, 242].

In the 1930s and 1940s, dithiocarbamates such as dimethyldithiocarbamates and diethyldithiocarbamates were used as pesticides against fungal pathogens on different crops [243], besides biocides in household products [244].

The industry plant physician E. E. Williams in 1937 observed that workers using tetramethylthiuram monosulfide and disulfide to facilitate the rubber vulcanization became alcohol-intolerant and quit consuming alcoholic beverages. The DSF-induced alcohol aversion was described in 1948 [245]. At that time, DSF was approached as a vermicide and employed as an ointment to treat scabies.

Afterward, besides alcoholism, DSF started to be studied for heavy metal poisoning, cancer [246–249], HIV [243, 250], as well as cocaine dependence, pathological gambling, and other psychiatric disorders [239] and other form of addiction, for example, the d-methamphetamine abuse [251]. Further tests are being performed focusing applications such as Alzheimer's disease [252], Lyme disease and babesiosis [253], tuberculosis [254], non-tuberculous mycobacteria infections [255], giardiasis [256], amoebiasis [257], obesity [258] and to revert drug resistance in different types of cancer [259–261], tuberculosis [262] bacterial infections [263], mycosis [264], giardiasis [265], etc. The repositioning of low-cost drugs such as DS is considered a "salvation" for global healthcare system [266].

Sodium diethylcarbamodithioate (**Figure 2**) (DETC also known as sodium (diethylcarbamothioyl)sulfanide; CAS no. 148-18-5; Molecular Formula: $C_5H_{11}NS_2.Na$) is the first derivative of DSF, involved in many of the biological activities of the latter.

Seemingly DETC is less toxic than aspirin [243], widely used, and well tolerated in humans [267] for decades being used up to 800 mg/twice/week, with no adverse effects [268]. DETC also known as Imuthiol or Dithiocarb was used as immunomodulator with good results on AIDS patients [269, 270] and was clinically employed in chronic bronchitis, rheumatoid arthritis, tuberculosis, and chronic infection [271].

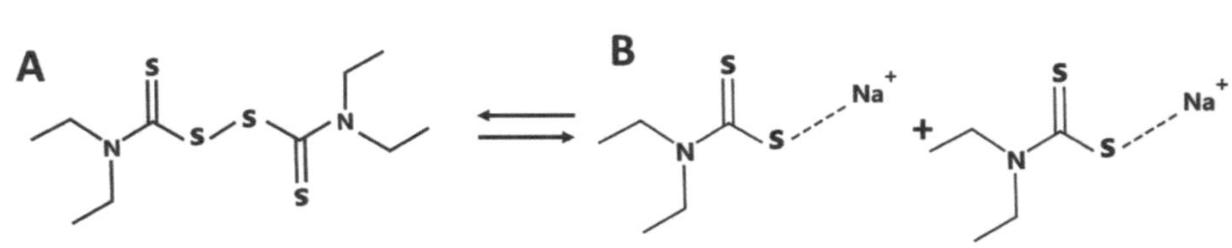


**Figure 2.**
*Molecular structures of disulfiram (A) and sodium diethyldithiocarbamate (B).*

In a seminal report on its antiparasitic activity, DETC was demonstrated to be leishmanicidal [272]. Afterward, novel delivery systems were developed to optimize the leishmanicidal activity of DETC [273–275]. In this regard, novel drug delivery systems are also developed for DSF [276]. The data obtained on Leishmania amazonensis motivated us to move to CD, employing the repositioned drug DSF combined to the drug of first choice BZ. Tests on NFX are in progress.

It is worth remembering that CD pathophysiology is associated with oxidative stress (*vide supra*), and both DSF [277] and DETC [278] can act as antioxidants. In addition, modulation of oxidative stress comprises a valuable tool in heart disease therapeutics [279]. In addition, DSF has antimutagenic properties [280].

### 5.2 Disulfiram combined to benznidazole in Chagas disease

Both DSF and DETC have antiparasitic activity on *T. cruzi* [281, 282], but the effectivity was not pronounced.

In our study, the DSF-BZ combination is promising since the antagonism of SOD activity can enhance oxidative stress in cancer cells [249] and *T. cruzi* [283]. In this regard, the antitumor activity of NTX is enhanced by SOD1 inhibition mediated by tetrathiomolybdate [284]. Both in vitro and in vivo experimental data confirmed the present assumption [Almeida-Silva et al., in press]. The SOD inhibition as well as TSH reaction by DSF/DETC can promote the intracellular accumulation of ROS leading to parasite death (**Figure 3**).

CD etiological therapy is often associated to severe adverse effects caused by the highly toxic drugs (*vide supra*). In this sense, the present innovation involves the advantage of employing DSF/DETC with cytoprotective properties [243] in different cell types.

DSF/DETC have neuroprotective [285], hepatoprotective [277], and nephroprotective [286] and even radioprotective [287, 288] activity. These protective effects may be beneficial in the treatment of parasitic diseases, because in the treatment of experimental infection by *T. rhodesiense*, DSF has marked protective activity (disulfiram rescue) against the toxic effects of diaminodichloroplatin and preventing the death of the treated organism [289].

Thus, the development of low-toxicity therapies may be expected, as DSF may have a protective action against the toxic effects of drugs such as cyclophosphamide [290], ifosfamide [291], N-nitrosodimethylamine [292], isoniazid [293] and the toxicity of α-naphthylisothiocyanate [294], acetaminophen [295], pyrrolizidines [296], the lethal effects of hypoxia [297], ischemia [298], as well as lead [299], cadmium [300], mercury, and other heavy metals [301]. Thus, DSF combinations can enable the development of safe medicines. Regarding CD, the cardioprotective and antioxidant activities of DSF/DETC as well as atrial neuroprotection [302] are particularly desirable [303–306]. In addition, DSF is effective as prophylactics in experimental colitis [307].

As drug resistance limits the successful CD therapy, the *T. cruzi* PgP expression has a pivotal role [308]. Therefore, it is relevant in the present approach that DSF/DETC inhibit PgP [261, 309, 310], causing the BZ accumulation within the parasite cytoplasm, enhancing trypanocidal activity, potentially reversing resistance phenotypes, such as $MDR^+$ (**Figure 3**). Interestingly, the ABCC proteins from *T. cruzi* are involved in thiol transport [311]. In view of the glutathione-drug adduct transport by ABC transporters (*vide supra*), it is interesting that DSF reduces GSH levels [54] at least in part through the formation of complexes with its different derivatives [312].

DSF [313] affects the redox balance of the cell, to GSH oxidation [314], reducing GSH levels [54] at least in part through the formation of complexes with its different

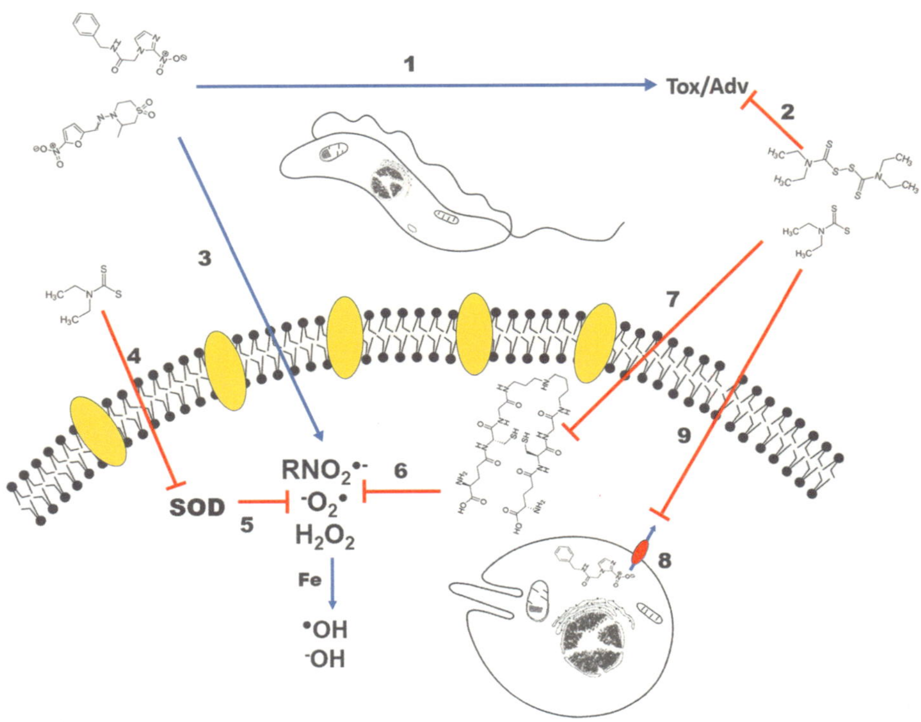


**Figure 3.**
*Putative mechanisms of action of disulfiram (DSF) or diethyldithiocarbamate (DETC) in combination with trypanocides in T. cruzi infection. Benznidazole (BZ) and nifurtimox are toxic and produce adverse reactions (1), which are ameliorated via detoxification mediated by DSF or DETC (2). The anti-T. cruzi agents trigger the formation of reactive oxygen species (ROS, 3) via nitroanion radicals ($RNO_2^{\bullet-}$) that give rise to superoxide ($O_2^{\bullet-}$), that is detoxified by superoxide dismutase (SOD, 5), generating hydrogen peroxide ($H_2O_2$), which in the presence of iron can produce hydroxyl radicals ($^\bullet OH$) and hydroxide anions ($^-OH$) via Fenton reaction. DETC inhibits SOD (4). ROS may be detoxified by reaction with sulfhydryl or thiol groups of trypanothione (N1,N8-bis(glutathionyl)spermidine, 6), and this adduct can be removed by reaction with thiols of DSF/DETC (7). The BZ molecules in the parasite cytoplasm are extruded from the cell via p-glycoproteins or MDR transporters (8), which are inhibited by DETC (9), presumably reversing resistance phenotypes.*

derivatives [312, 315]. DETC can also reduce the GSH/non-protein thiol levels, also leading to the reduction of glutathione peroxidase activities [53, 316].

The combinations tested here may also contribute to resistance reversal, also through DETC-mediated inhibition of Fe-dependent SOD, which is linked to resistance to BZ in *T. cruzi* [66, 162, 163].

Furthermore, DSF can be used against cancer cells targeting the ubiquitin-proteasome system [317], and the ubiquitin-proteasome pathway is a therapeutic target in *T. cruzi* [318].

In this way, the strategy based of combinations of the repositioned drugs proposed here can achieve effectiveness, with selectivity and, therefore, safety in the CD treatment and sheds new light on perspectives for new therapeutic strategies.

## 6. The clinical stage

Translational research in biomedical sciences translates basic research and experimental discoveries into health taking the route from benchtop to bedside. This important field has gained substantial attention and investments in the last two decades [319].

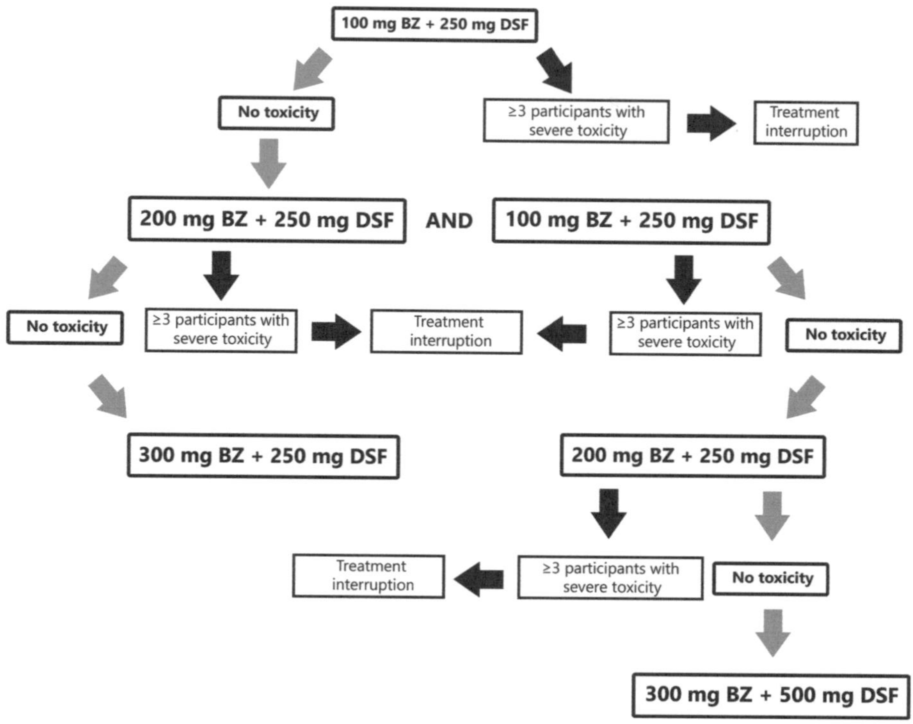


**Figure 4.**
*Design of the clinical trial for testing the BZ-DSF combination. Reproduced from Ref. [320] (with permission).*

In order to reach a proof of concept on the effectivity of the DSF-BZ combination in human infection, a partnership was established gathering different units of Fiocruz. The present study comprises a translational approach that began with experiments in vitro, on the bench and now reaches the clinical stage at the Evandro Chagas National Institute of Infectious Diseases-Fiocruz, coordinated by the team of the Clinical Research Laboratory of Chagas Disease, with assistance of the Clinical Research platform. Therefore, the phase I/II clinical trial was elaborated (**Figure 4**) and published recently [320].

## 7. Conclusions and future perspectives

The use of DSF/DETC combined to BZ in CD treatment comprises a potential innovative therapeutical tool, possibly overcoming adverse reactions and refractory cases. Since these repositioned drugs exert cytoprotective effects, reducing the adverse reactions of many drugs, safe combinations can be potentially identified, leading to the development of well-tolerated medication. Therefore, therapy interruption can be precluded, consequently increasing patient adherence. In addition, as DSF/DETC can inhibit p-glycoprotein activity as well as reduce GSH levels, two molecules involved in drug extrusion from $MDR^+$ parasites, it is reasonable to suppose the combination could eventually revert/downmodulate natural/acquired resistance phenotypes. Thus, treatment may be effective even in refractory cases. We are now approaching the clinical response of chronic phase CD patients. A possible proof of concept may lead to the development of a safe and effective medication, with profound implications in treatment prognosis, presumably improving the quality of life of the patients.

## Acknowledgements

This research was sponsored by grants from the Conselho Nacional de Desenvolvimento Científico e Tecnológico (CNPq grant no. 443886/2018-0 to RMS and CNPq grant no. 314717/2020 to MAVS), Fundação Carlos Chagas Filho de Amparo à Pesquisa do Rio de Janeiro (FAPERJ grant no. 211.167/2019 to RMS; FAPERJ grant no. 260475/2021 and 259286/2021 to MAVS and FAPERJ grant no. 204.388/2021 to AMSF) and Fundação Oswaldo Cruz (Fiocruz grant no. 6221125199 to MAVS).

## Author details

Marcos André Vannier-Santos[1*], Ana Márcia Suarez-Fontes[1], Juliana Almeida-Silva[1], Alessandra Lifsitch Viçosa[2], Sandra Aurora Chavez Perez[2], Alejandro Marcel Hasslocher-Moreno[3], Gabriel Parreiras Estolano da Silveira[4], Luciana Fernandes Portela[3] and Roberto Magalhães Saraiva[3]

1 Laboratory of Innovations on Therapies, Education and Bioproducts (LITEB), Oswaldo Cruz Institute, Oswaldo Cruz Foundation (IOC-FIOCRUZ), Rio de Janeiro, Brazil

2 Institute of Technology in Drugs, Oswaldo Cruz Foundation (Farmanguinhos/FIOCRUZ), Rio de Janeiro, Brazil

3 Clinical Research Laboratory of Chagas Disease (Lapclin-Chagas), Evandro Chagas National Institute of Infectious Diseases, Oswaldo Cruz Foundation (INI-FIOCRUZ), Rio de Janeiro, Brazil

4 Pharmacodynamics Service, Oswaldo Cruz Foundation (FIOCRUZ), Rio de Janeiro, Brazil

*Address all correspondence to: marcos.vannier@ioc.fiocruz.br; marcos.vannier@pesquisador.cnpq.br

## References

[1] Schmunis GA, Yadon ZE. Chagas disease: A Latin American health problem becoming a world health problem. Acta Tropica. 2010;**115**(1-2): 14-21

[2] Montgomery SP, Parise ME, Dotson EM, Bialek SR. What do we know about Chagas disease in the United States? The American Journal of Tropical Medicine and Hygiene. 2016;**95**(6):1225-1227

[3] Harris N, Woc-Colburn L, Gunter SM, Gorchakov R, Murray KO, Rossmann S, et al. Autochthonous Chagas disease in the Southern United States: A case report of suspected residential and military exposures. Zoonoses and Public Health. 2017;**64**(6):491-493

[4] Lynn MK, Bossak BH, Sandifer PA, Watson A, Nolan MS. Contemporary autochthonous human Chagas disease in the USA. Acta Tropica. 2020;**205**:105361

[5] Rowland ME, Maloney J, Cohen S, Yabsley MJ, Huang J, Kranz M, et al. Factors associated with *Trypanosoma cruzi* exposure among domestic Canines in Tennessee. The Journal of Parasitology. 2010;**96**(3):547-551

[6] Thompson JM, Habrun CA, Scully CM, Sasaki E, Bauer RW, Jania R, et al. Locally transmitted *Trypanosoma cruzi* in a Domestic Llama (*Lama glama*) in a rural area of Greater New Orleans, Louisiana, USA. Vector Borne and Zoonotic Diseases. 2021;**21**(10):762-768

[7] Busselman RE, Hamer SA. Chagas Disease Ecology in the United States: Recent Advances in Understanding *Trypanosoma cruzi* Transmission Among Triatomines, Wildlife, and Domestic Animals and a Quantitative Synthesis of Vector-Host Interactions. Annual Review of Animal Biosciences. 2022;**10**:325-348

[8] Busselman RE, Meyers AC, Zecca IB, Auckland LD, Castro AH, Dowd RE, et al. High incidence of *Trypanosoma cruzi* infections in dogs directly detected through longitudinal tracking at 10 multi-dog kennels, Texas, USA. PLoS Neglected Tropical Diseases. 2021;**15**(11):e0009935

[9] Coura JR, Viñas PA. Chagas disease: A new worldwide challenge. Nature. 2010;**465**(S7301):S6-S7

[10] Franco-Paredes C, Bottazzi ME, Hotez PJ. The unfinished public health agenda of Chagas disease in the era of globalization. PLoS Neglected Tropical Diseases. 2009;**3**(7):e470

[11] Parker ER, Sethi A. Chagas disease: Coming to a place near you. Dermatologic Clinics. 2011;**29**(1):53-62

[12] Garza M, Feria Arroyo TP, Casillas EA, Sanchez-Cordero V, Rivaldi C-L, Sarkar S. Projected future distributions of vectors of *Trypanosoma cruzi* in North America under climate change scenarios. PLoS Neglected Tropical Diseases. 2014;**8**(5):e2818

[13] Eberhard FE, Cunze S, Kochmann J, Klimpel S. Modelling the climatic suitability of Chagas disease vectors on a global scale. eLife. 2020;**6**(9):e52072

[14] Telleria J, Tibayrenc M. American Trypanosomiasis: Chagas Disease One Hundred Years of Research. 1st ed. Amsterdam: Elsevier; 2010. 844 p

[15] Dias JP, Bastos C, Araújo E, Mascarenhas AV, Martins Netto E,

Grassi F, et al. Acute Chagas disease outbreak associated with oral transmission. Revista da Sociedade Brasileira de Medicina Tropical. 2008;**41**(3):296-300

[16] de Noya B, González O, Robertson LJ. *Trypanosoma cruzi* as a Foodborne Pathogen. Cham: Springer International Publishing; 2015

[17] Suárez DC, Rey ÁP, Orduz ML, Prada RL, Tarazona Z. Survival of *Trypanosoma cruzi* in experimentally contaminated drinks. Biomédica. 2016;**32**(1):134-148

[18] WHO (World Health Organization). Chagas Disease (American trypanosomiasis). 2018

[19] Carlos Pinto Dias J, Novaes Ramos A, Dias Gontijo E, Luquetti A, Aparecida Shikanai-Yasuda M, Rodrigues Coura J, et al. II Consenso Brasileiro em Doença de Chagas, 2015. Epidemiologia e Serviços de Saúde. 2016;**25**(21):1-10

[20] Araujo-Jorge TC, Ferreira RR, Rocha RCM, Vieira TM, Costa ND, Santos LL, et al. "Chagas Express XXI": A new ArtScience social technology for health and science education—A case study in Brazilian endemic areas of Chagas disease with an active search of chronic cases. PLoS Neglected Tropical Diseases. 2021;**15**(7):e0009534

[21] Lee BY, Bacon KM, Bottazzi ME, Hotez PJ. Global economic burden of Chagas disease: A computational simulation model. The Lancet Infectious Diseases. 2013;**13**(4):342-348

[22] PAHO (Pan American Health Organization). Chagas disease. 2019

[23] Urbina JA. Specific chemotherapy of Chagas disease: Relevance, current limitations and new approaches. Acta Tropica. 2010;**115**(1-2):55-68

[24] Bartel LC, Montalto de Mecca M, Fanelli SL, Rodriguez de Castro C, Diaz EG, Castro JA. Early nifurtimox-induced biochemical and ultrastructural alterations in rat heart. Human & Experimental Toxicology. 2007;**26**(10):781-788

[25] de Mecca MM, Fanelli SL, Bartel LC, de Castro CR, Díaz EG, Castro JA. Nifurtimox nitroreductase activity in different cellular fractions from male rat pancreas. Biochemical and ultrastructural alterations. Life Sciences. 2007;**81**(2):144-152

[26] Mecca MM de, Bartel LC, Castro CR de, Castro JA. Benznidazole biotransformation in rat heart microsomal fraction without observable ultrastructural alterations: Comparison to Nifurtimox-induced cardiac effects. Memórias do Instituto Oswaldo Cruz 2008;**103**(6):549-553

[27] Vannier-Santos M, De Castro S. Electron microscopy in antiparasitic chemotherapy: A (close) view to a kill. Current Drug Targets. 2009;**10**(3):246-260

[28] Vannier-Santos MA, Brunoro GV, Soeiro MN, DeCastro SL, Menna-Barreto FS. Parasite, Compartments, and Molecules: Trick versus Treatment on Chagas Disease. In: De Souza W, editor. Biology of *Trypanosoma cruzi*. 1st ed. London, UK: IntechOpen; 2019

[29] Menna-Barreto RFS. Cell death pathways in pathogenic trypanosomatids: Lessons of (over)kill. Cell Death & Disease. 2019;**10**(2):93

[30] Castro JA, Diaz de Toranzo EG. Toxic effects of nifurtimox and benznidazole, two drugs used against American

trypanosomiasis (Chagas' disease). Biomedical and Environmental Sciences. 1988;**1**(1):19-33

[31] Castro JA, DeMecca MM, Bartel LC. Toxic side effects of drugs used to treat Chagas' disease (American trypanosomiasis). Human & Experimental Toxicology. 2006;**25**(8): 471-479

[32] Pérez-Molina JA, Crespillo-Andújar C, Bosch-Nicolau P, Molina I. Trypanocidal treatment of Chagas disease. Enfermedades Infecciosas y Microbiología Clínica. 2021;**39**(9):458-470

[33] Jackson Y, Wyssa B, Chappuis F. Tolerance to nifurtimox and benznidazole in adult patients with chronic Chagas' disease. The Journal of Antimicrobial Chemotherapy. 2020;**75**(3):690-696

[34] Olivera MJ, Cucunubá ZM, Álvarez CA, Nicholls RS. Safety profile of nifurtimox and treatment interruption for chronic Chagas disease in Colombian adults. The American Journal of Tropical Medicine and Hygiene. 2015;**93**(6):1224-1230

[35] Olivera MJ, Cucunubá ZM, Valencia-Hernández CA, Herazo R, Agreda-Rudenko D, Flórez C, et al. Risk factors for treatment interruption and severe adverse effects to benznidazole in adult patients with Chagas disease. PLoS One. 2017;**12**(9):e0185033

[36] Sperandio da Silva GM, Mediano MFF, da Costa Chambela M, da Silva JA, de Sousa AS, Alvarenga Americano do Brasil PE. A clinical adverse drug reaction prediction model for patients with Chagas disease treated with benznidazole. Antimicrobial Agents and Chemotherapy. 2014;**58**(11):6371-6377

[37] Hasslocher-Moreno AM, do Brasil PE, de Sousa AS, Xavier SS, Chambela MC, Sperandio da Silva GM. Safety of benznidazole use in the treatment of chronic Chagas' disease. The Journal of Antimicrobial Chemotherapy. 2012;**67**(5):1261-1266

[38] Levi GC, Lobo IMF, Kallás EG, Amato NV. Etiological drug treatment of human infection by *Trypanosoma cruzi*. Revista do Instituto de Medicina Tropical de São Paulo. 1996;**38**(1):35-38

[39] Crespillo-Andújar C, López-Vélez R, Trigo E, Norman F, Díaz-Menéndez M, Monge-Maillo B, et al. Comparison of the toxicity of two treatment schemes with benznidazole for chronic Chagas disease: A prospective cohort study in two Spanish referral centres. Clinical Microbiology and Infection. 2020;**26**(3):384

[40] Guggenbühl Noller JM, Froeschl G, Eisermann P, Jochum J, Theuring S, Reiter-Owona I, et al. Describing nearly two decades of Chagas disease in Germany and the lessons learned: A retrospective study on screening, detection, diagnosis, and treatment of *Trypanosoma cruzi* infection from 2000-2018. BMC Infectious Diseases. 2020;**20**(1):919

[41] Pérez-Molina JA, Sojo-Dorado J, Norman F, Monge-Maillo B, Díaz-Menéndez M, Albajar-Viñas P, et al. Nifurtimox therapy for Chagas disease does not cause hypersensitivity reactions in patients with such previous adverse reactions during benznidazole treatment. Acta Tropica. 2013;**127**(2):101-104

[42] Pérez-Molina JA, Molina I. Chagas disease. Lancet. 2018;**391**(10115):82-94

[43] Viotti R, Vigliano C, Armenti H, Segura E. Treatment of chronic Chagas' disease with benznidazole: Clinical and

serologic evolution of patients with long-term follow-up. American Heart Journal. 1994;**127**(1):151-162

[44] Hasslocher-Moreno AM, Saraiva RM, Sangenis LHC, Xavier SS, de Sousa AS, Costa AR, et al. Benznidazole decreases the risk of chronic Chagas disease progression and cardiovascular events: A long-term follow up study. eClinicalMedicine. 2021;**31**:100694

[45] Urbina JA. Parasitological cure of Chagas disease: Is it possible? Is it relevant? Memórias do Instituto Oswaldo Cruz. 1999;**94**(Suppl. 1):349-355

[46] Cal M, Ioset J-R, Fügi MA, Mäser P, Kaiser M. Assessing anti-*T. cruzi* candidates in vitro for sterile cidality. International Journal for Parasitology: Drugs and Drug Resistance. 2016;**6**(3):165-170

[47] Neal RA, van Bueren J. Comparative studies of drug susceptibility of five strains of *Trypanosoma cruzi* in vivo and in vitro. Transactions of the Royal Society of Tropical Medicine and Hygiene. 1988;**82**(5):709-714

[48] Lin C, Ferreira de Almeida Fiuza L, Cardoso Santos C, Ferreira Nunes D, Cruz Moreira O, Bouton J, et al. 6-Methyl-7-aryl-7-deazapurine nucleosides as anti-*Trypanosoma cruzi* agents: Structure-activity relationship and in vivo efficacy. ChemMedChem. 2021;**16**(14):2231-2253

[49] Pinazo M-J, Espinosa G, Cortes-Lletget C, Posada E, Aldasoro E, Oliveira I, et al. Immunosuppression and Chagas disease: A management challenge. PLoS Neglected Tropical Diseases. 2013;**7**(1):e1965

[50] Sánchez-Valdéz FJ, Padilla A, Wang W, Orr D, Tarleton RL. Spontaneous dormancy protects *Trypanosoma cruzi* during extended drug exposure. eLife. 2018;**26**(7):e34039

[51] Barrett MP, Kyle DE, Sibley LD, Radke JB, Tarleton RL. Protozoan persister-like cells and drug treatment failure. Nature Reviews. Microbiology. 2019;**17**(10):607-620

[52] Nagajyothi F, Machado FS, Burleigh BA, Jelicks LA, Scherer PE, Mukherjee S, et al. Mechanisms of *Trypanosoma cruzi* persistence in Chagas disease. Cellular Microbiology. 2012;**14**(5):634-643

[53] Strömme JH. Effects of diethyldithiocarbamate and disulfiram on glucose metabolism and glutathione content of human erythrocytes. Biochemical Pharmacology. 1963;**12**(7):705-715

[54] Mittal M, Khan K, Pal S, Porwal K, China SP, Barbhuyan TK, et al. The thiocarbamate disulphide drug, disulfiram induces osteopenia in rats by inhibition of osteoblast function due to suppression of acetaldehyde dehydrogenase activity. Toxicological Sciences. 2014;**139**(1):257-270

[55] Heikkila RE, Cabbat FS, Cohen G. Inactivation of superoxide dismutase by several thiocarbamic acid derivatives. Experientia. 1978;**34**(12):1553-1554

[56] Heikkila RE, Cabbat FS, Cohen G. In vivo inhibition of superoxide dismutase in mice by diethyldithiocarbamate. The Journal of Biological Chemistry. 1976;**251**(7):2182-2185

[57] Doyon G, Zerbato J, Mellors JW, Sluis-Cremer N. Disulfiram reactivates latent HIV-1 expression through depletion of the phosphatase and tensin homolog. AIDS. 2013;**27**(2):F7-F11

[58] Kim Y, Anderson JL, Lewin SR. Getting the "Kill" into "Shock and Kill":

Strategies to eliminate latent HIV. Cell Host & Microbe. 2018;**23**(1):14-26

[59] Maeda FY, Cortez C, Yoshida N. Cell signaling during *Trypanosoma cruzi* invasion. Frontiers in Immunology. 2012;**3**:361

[60] Burleigh BA, Woolsey AM. Cell signalling and *Trypanosoma cruzi* invasion. Cellular Microbiology. 2002;**4**(11):701-711

[61] Chuenkova MV, Furnari FB, Cavenee WK, Pereira MA. *Trypanosoma cruzi* trans-sialidase: A potent and specific survival factor for human Schwann cells by means of phosphatidylinositol 3-kinase/Akt signaling. Proceedings of the National Academy of Sciences. 2001;**98**(17):9936-9941

[62] Zhang H, Chen D, Ringler J, Chen W, Cui QC, Ethier SP, et al. Disulfiram treatment facilitates phosphoinositide 3-kinase inhibition in human breast cancer cells in vitro and in vivo. Cancer Research. 2010;**70**(10):3996-4004

[63] Bustamante JM, Sanchez-Valdez F, Padilla AM, White B, Wang W, Tarleton RL. A modified drug regimen clears active and dormant trypanosomes in mouse models of Chagas disease. Science Translational Medicine. 2020;**12**(567):eabb7656

[64] Pessenda G, Silva JS. Arginase and its mechanisms in Leishmania persistence. Parasite Immunology. 2020;**42**(7):e12722

[65] Mejia AM, Hall BS, Taylor MC, Gómez-Palacio A, Wilkinson SR, Triana-Chávez O, et al. Benznidazole-resistance in *Trypanosoma cruzi* is a readily acquired trait that can arise independently in a single population. The Journal of Infectious Diseases. 2012;**206**(2):220-228

[66] Campos MCO, Leon LL, Taylor MC, Kelly JM. Benznidazole-resistance in *Trypanosoma cruzi*: Evidence that distinct mechanisms can act in concert. Molecular and Biochemical Parasitology. 2014;**193**(1):17-19

[67] Francisco AF, Jayawardhana S, Olmo F, Lewis MD, Wilkinson SR, Taylor MC, et al. Challenges in Chagas disease drug development. Molecules. 2020;**25**(12):2799

[68] Filardi LS, Brener Z. Susceptibility and natural resistance of *Trypanosoma cruzi* strains to drugs used clinically in Chagas disease. Transactions of the Royal Society of Tropical Medicine and Hygiene. 1987;**81**(5):755-759

[69] Zingales B. *Trypanosoma cruzi* genetic diversity: Something new for something known about Chagas disease manifestations, serodiagnosis and drug sensitivity. Acta Tropica. 2018; **184**:38-52

[70] Teston APM, Monteiro WM, Reis D, Bossolani GDP, Gomes ML, de Araújo SM, et al. In vivo susceptibility to benznidazole of *Trypanosoma cruzi* strains from the western Brazilian Amazon. Tropical Medicine & International Health. 2013;**18**(1):85-95

[71] Zingales B, Araujo RGA, Moreno M, Franco J, Aguiar PHN, Nunes SL, et al. A novel ABCG-like transporter of *Trypanosoma cruzi* is involved in natural resistance to benznidazole. Memórias do Instituto Oswaldo Cruz. 2015;**110**(3):433-444

[72] Loffredo L, Violi F. COVID-19 and cardiovascular injury: A role for oxidative stress and antioxidant treatment? International Journal of Cardiology. 2020;**312**:136

[73] Dichi I, Breganó JW, Simão ANC, Cecchini R. Role of Oxidative Stress in

Chronic Diseases. 1st ed. Boca Raton: CRC Press; 2014. 720 p

[74] Bondy SC, Campbell A. Inflammation, aging, and oxidative stress. In: Bondy SC, Campbell A, editors. Oxidative Stress in Applied Basic Research and Clinical Practice. Cham: Springer International Publishing; 2016

[75] Armstrong D, Stratton RD. Oxidative Stress and Antioxidant Protection: The Science of Free Radical Biology and Disease. 1st ed. Hoboken, New Jersey: John Wiley & Sons Inc.; 2016. 600 p

[76] Sies H. (Ed.). Oxidative stress: eustress and distress. London: Academic Press; 2020. 829 p

[77] Lushchak V, Semchyshyn H, editors. Oxidative Stress: Molecular Mechanisms and Biological Effects. London, UK: InTechOpen; 2012

[78] Flohé L. Glutathione. Boca Raton: Taylor & Francis; 2018

[79] Piñeyro MD, Arias D, Parodi-Talice A, Guerrero S, Robello C. Trypanothione metabolism as drug target for trypanosomatids. Current Pharmaceutical Design. 2021;**27**(15): 1834-1846

[80] Fairlamb AH, Cerami A. Metabolism and functions of trypanothione in the kinetoplastida. Annual Review of Microbiology. 1992;**46**(1):695-729

[81] Pountain AW, Weidt SK, Regnault C, Bates PA, Donachie AM, Dickens NJ, et al. Genomic instability at the locus of sterol C24-methyltransferase promotes amphotericin B resistance in Leishmania parasites. PLoS Neglected Tropical Diseases. 2019;**13**(2):e0007052

[82] Ozols RF, O'Dwyer PJ, Hamilton TC, Young RC. The role of glutathione in drug resistance. Cancer Treatment Reviews. 1990;**17**:45-50

[83] Schröder CP, Godwin AK, O'Dwyer PJ, Tew KD, Hamilton TC, Ozols RF. Glutathione and drug resistance. Cancer Investigation. 1996;**14**(2):158-168

[84] Russell TM, Azad MG, Richardson DR. The relationship of glutathione-S-transferase and multi-drug resistance-related protein 1 in nitric oxide (NO) transport and storage. Molecules. 2021;**26**(19):5784

[85] Moncada C, Repetto Y, Aldunate J, Letelier ME, Morello A. Role of glutathione in the susceptibility of *Trypanosoma cruzi* to drugs. Comparative Biochemistry and Physiology - Part C. 1989;**94**(1):87-91

[86] Repetto Y, Opazo E, Maya JD, Agosin M, Morello A. Glutathione and trypanothione in several strains of *Trypanosoma cruzi*: Effect of drugs. Comparative Biochemistry and Physiology, Part B: Biochemistry & Molecular Biology. 1996;**115**(2):281-285

[87] Mesías AC, Sasoni N, Arias DG, Pérez Brandán C, Orban OCF, Kunick C, et al. Trypanothione synthetase confers growth, survival advantage and resistance to anti-protozoal drugs in *Trypanosoma cruzi*. Free Radical Biology & Medicine. 2019;**130**:23-34

[88] Faúndez M, Pino L, Letelier P, Ortiz C, López R, Seguel C, et al. Buthionine sulfoximine increases the toxicity of nifurtimox and benznidazole to *Trypanosoma cruzi*. Antimicrobial Agents and Chemotherapy. 2005;**49**(1):126-130

[89] Faúndez M, López-Muñoz R, Torres G, Morello A, Ferreira J, Kemmerling U, et al. Buthionine

sulfoximine has anti-*Trypanosoma cruzi* activity in a murine model of acute Chagas' disease and enhances the efficacy of nifurtimox. Antimicrobial Agents and Chemotherapy. 2008;**52**(5):1837-1839

[90] Carter KC, Sundar S, Spickett C, Pereira OC, Mullen AB. The in vivo susceptibility of *Leishmania donovani* to sodium stibogluconate is drug specific and can be reversed by inhibiting glutathione biosynthesis. Antimicrobial Agents and Chemotherapy. 2003;**47**(5): 1529-1535

[91] Vannier-Santos MA, Suarez-Fontes AM. Role of polyamines in parasite cell architecture and function. Current Pharmaceutical Design. 2017;**23**(23):3342-3358

[92] Phillips MA. Polyamines in protozoan pathogens. The Journal of Biological Chemistry. 2018;**293**(48):18746-18756

[93] Hernández SM, Sánchez MS, de Tarlovsky MNS. Polyamines as a defense mechanism against lipoperoxidation in *Trypanosoma cruzi*. Acta Tropica. 2006;**98**(1):94-102

[94] Birkholtz L-M, Williams M, Niemand J, Louw AI, Persson L, Heby O. Polyamine homoeostasis as a drug target in pathogenic protozoa: Peculiarities and possibilities. The Biochemical Journal. 2011;**438**(2):229-244

[95] Roberts S, Ullman B. Parasite polyamines as pharmaceutical targets. Current Pharmaceutical Design. 2017;**23**(23):3325-3341

[96] Talevi A, Carrillo C, Comini M. The thiol-polyamine metabolism of *Trypanosoma cruzi*: Molecular targets and drug repurposing strategies. Current Medicinal Chemistry. 2019;**26**(36):6614-6635

[97] de Oliveira TB, Pedrosa RC, Filho DW. Oxidative stress in chronic cardiopathy associated with Chagas disease. International Journal of Cardiology. 2007;**116**(3):357-363

[98] Gupta S, Wen J-J, Garg NJ. Oxidative sress in Chagas disease. Interdisciplinary Perspectives on Infectious Diseases. 2009;**2009**:1-8

[99] Zacks MA, Wen J-J, Vyatkina G, Bhatia V, Garg N. An overview of chagasic cardiomyopathy: Pathogenic importance of oxidative stress. Anais da Academia Brasileira de Ciências. 2005;**77**(4):695-715

[100] Wen J, Yachelini PC, Sembaj A, Manzur RE, Garg NJ. Increased oxidative stress is correlated with mitochondrial dysfunction in chagasic patients. Free Radical Biology & Medicine. 2006;**41**(2):270-276

[101] Turrens JF. Superoxide production by the mitochondrial respiratory chain. Bioscience Reports. 1997;**17**(1):3-8

[102] Turrens JF. Mitochondrial formation of reactive oxygen species. The Journal of Physiology. 2003;**552**(2):335-344

[103] Prolo C, Estrada D, Piacenza L, Benítez D, Comini MA, Radi R, et al. Nox2-derived superoxide radical is crucial to control acute *Trypanosoma cruzi* infection. Redox Biology. 2021;**46**:102085

[104] Wen J-J, Garg N. Oxidative modification of mitochondrial respiratory complexes in response to the stress of *Trypanosoma cruzi* infection. Free Radical Biology & Medicine. 2004;**37**(12):2072-2081

[105] Dhiman M, Wan X, Popov VL, Vargas G, Garg NJ. MnSOD tg mice control myocardial inflammatory

and oxidative stress and remodeling responses elicited in chronic Chagas disease. Journal of the American Heart Association. 2013;**2**(5):e000302

[106] Maldonado E, Rojas DA, Morales S, Miralles V, Solari A. Dual and opposite roles of reactive oxygen species (ROS) in Chagas disease: Beneficial on the pathogen and harmful on the host. Oxidative Medicine and Cellular Longevity. 2020;**2020**:1-17

[107] Maldonado E, Rojas DA, Urbina F, Solari A. The oxidative stress and chronic inflammatory process in Chagas disease: Role of exosomes and contributing genetic factors. Oxidative Medicine and Cellular Longevity. 2021;**2021**:1-21

[108] Wen J-J, Vyatkina G, Garg N. Oxidative damage during chagasic cardiomyopathy development: Role of mitochondrial oxidant release and inefficient antioxidant defense. Free Radical Biology & Medicine. 2004;**37**(11):1821-1833

[109] Dantas-Pereira L, Menna-Barreto R, Lannes-Vieira J. Extracellular vesicles: Potential role in remote signaling and inflammation in Trypanosoma cruzi triggered disease. Frontiers in Cell and Development Biology. 2021;**9**:798054

[110] Chuenkova MV, Pereiraperrin M. Neurodegeneration and neuroregeneration in Chagas disease. Advances in Parasitology. 2011;**76**:195-233

[111] Vilar-Pereira G, Castaño Barrios L, Silva AA, Martins Batista A, Resende Pereira I, Cruz Moreira O, et al. Memory impairment in chronic experimental Chagas disease: Benznidazole therapy reversed cognitive deficit in association with reduction of parasite load and oxidative stress in the nervous tissue. PLoS One. 2021;**16**(1):e0244710

[112] Wen J-J, Garg NJ. Mitochondrial generation of reactive oxygen species is enhanced at the Qo site of the complex III in the myocardium of *Trypanosoma cruzi*-infected mice: Beneficial effects of an antioxidant. Journal of Bioenergetics and Biomembranes. 2008;**40**(6):587-598

[113] Sánchez-Villamil JP, Bautista-Niño PK, Serrano NC, Rincon MY, Garg NJ. Potential role of antioxidants as adjunctive therapy in Chagas disease. Oxidative Medicine and Cellular Longevity. 2020;**2020**:1-13

[114] Du J, Cullen JJ, Buettner GR. Ascorbic acid: Chemistry, biology and the treatment of cancer. Biochimica et Biophysica Acta, Reviews on Cancer. 2012;**1826**(2):443-457

[115] Mastrangelo D, Pelosi E, Castelli G, Lo-Coco F, Testa U. Mechanisms of anti-cancer effects of ascorbate: Cytotoxic activity and epigenetic modulation. Blood Cells, Molecules & Diseases. 2018;**69**:57-64

[116] Puente V, Demaria A, Frank FM, Batlle A, Lombardo ME. Anti-parasitic effect of vitamin C alone and in combination with benznidazole against *Trypanosoma cruzi*. PLoS Neglected Tropical Diseases. 2018;**12**(9):e0006764

[117] Providello MV, Carneiro ZA, Portapilla GB, do Vale GT, Camargo RS, Tirapelli CR, et al. Benefits of ascorbic acid in association with low-dose benznidazole in treatment of Chagas disease. Antimicrobial Agents and Chemotherapy. 2018;**62**(9):e00514-18

[118] Piacenza L, Trujillo M, Radi R. Reactive species and pathogen antioxidant networks during phagocytosis. The Journal of Experimental Medicine. 2019;**216**(3):501-516

[119] Piacenza L, Peluffo G, Alvarez MN, Martínez A, Radi R. *Trypanosoma cruzi* antioxidant enzymes as virulence factors in Chagas disease. Antioxidants & Redox Signaling. 2013;**19**(7):723-734

[120] Oyenihi OR, Oyenihi AB, Alabi TD, Tade OG, Adeyanju AA, Oguntibeju OO. Reactive oxygen species: Key players in the anticancer effects of apigenin? Journal of Food Biochemistry. 2022;**46**(2):e14060

[121] Goes GR, Rocha PS, Diniz ARS, Aguiar PHN, Machado CR, Vieira LQ. *Trypanosoma cruzi* needs a signal provided by reactive oxygen species to infect macrophages. PLoS Neglected Tropical Diseases. 2016;**10**(4):e0004555

[122] Paiva CN, Feijó DF, Dutra FF, Carneiro VC, Freitas GB, Alves LS, et al. Oxidative stress fuels *Trypanosoma cruzi* infection in mice. The Journal of Clinical Investigation. 2012;**122**(7):2531-2542

[123] Dumoulin PC, Burleigh BA. Stress induced proliferation and cell cycle plasticity of intracellular *Trypanosoma cruzi* amastigotes. MBio. 2018;**9**(4):e00673-18

[124] Batinić-Haberle I, Rebouças JS, Spasojević I. Redox-Active Therapeutics. 1st ed. Switzerland: Springer International Publishing; 2016. 1261 p

[125] Turrens JF. Oxidative stress and antioxidant defenses: A target for the treatment of diseases caused by parasitic protozoa. Molecular Aspects of Medicine. 2004;**25**(1-2):211-220

[126] Docampo R, Moreno SNJ. Free radical metabolites in the mode of action of chemotherapeutic agents and phagocytic cells on *Trypanosoma cruzi*. Clinical Infectious Diseases. 1984;**6**(2):223-238

[127] Beltran-Hortelano I, Perez-Silanes S, Galiano S. Trypanothione reductase and superoxide dismutase as current drug targets for *Trypanosoma cruzi*: An overview of compounds with activity against Chagas disease. Current Medicinal Chemistry. 2017;**24**(11):1066-1138

[128] Boveris A, Docampo R, Turrens JF, Stoppani AO. Effect of β-lapachone on superoxide anion and hydrogen peroxide production in *Trypanosoma cruzi*. The Biochemical Journal. 1978;**175**(2):431-439

[129] Cruz FS, Docampo R, de Souza W. Effect of beta-lapachone on hydrogen peroxide production in *Trypanosoma cruzi*. Acta Tropica. 1978;**35**(1):35-40

[130] Docampo R, Cruz FS, Boveris A, Muniz RPA, Esquivel DMS. Lipid peroxidation and the generation of free radicals, superoxide anion, and hydrogen peroxide in β-lapachone-treated *Trypanosoma cruzi* epimastigotes. Archives of Biochemistry and Biophysics. 1978;**186**(2):292-297

[131] Bombaça ACS, Viana PG, Santos ACC, Silva TL, Rodrigues ABM, Guimarães ACR, et al. Mitochondrial disfunction and ROS production are essential for anti-*Trypanosoma cruzi* activity of β-lapachone-derived naphthoimidazoles. Free Radical Biology & Medicine. 2019;**130**:408-418

[132] Gong Q, Hu J, Wang P, Li X, Zhang X. A comprehensive review on β-lapachone: Mechanisms, structural modifications, and therapeutic potentials. European Journal of Medicinal Chemistry. 2021;**210**: 112962

[133] Menna-BarretoRFS,Henriques-PonsA, Pinto AV, Morgado-Diaz JA, Soares MJ, De Castro SL. Effect of a β-lapachone-derived naphthoimidazole on *Trypanosoma cruzi*: Identification of target organelles. The Journal

of Antimicrobial Chemotherapy. 2005;**56**(6):1034-1041

[134] dos Anjos DO, Sobral Alves ES, Gonçalves VT, Fontes SS, Nogueira ML, Suarez-Fontes AM, et al. Effects of a novel β-lapachone derivative on *Trypanosoma cruzi*: Parasite death involving apoptosis, autophagy and necrosis. International Journal for Parasitology: Drugs and Drug Resistance. 2016;**6**(3):207-219

[135] Yang Y, Karakhanova S, Hartwig W, D'Haese JG, Philippov PP, Werner J, et al. Mitochondria and mitochondrial ROS in cancer: Novel targets for anticancer therapy. Journal of Cellular Physiology. 2016;**231**(12):2570-2581

[136] Dhote V, Samundre P, Ganeshpurkar A, Upaganlawar A. Aging of brain related with mitochondrial dysfunctions. Current Drug Targets. 2021;**22**(14):1668-1687

[137] Dabravolski SA, Nikiforov NG, Starodubova AV, Popkova TV, Orekhov AN. The role of mitochondria-derived peptides in cardiovascular diseases and their potential as therapeutic targets. International Journal of Molecular Sciences. 2021;**22**(16):8770

[138] Clayton SA, MacDonald L, Kurowska-Stolarska M, Clark AR. Mitochondria as key players in the pathogenesis and treatment of rheumatoid arthritis. Frontiers in Immunology. 2021;**12**:673916

[139] Sharma VK, Singh TG, Mehta V. Stressed mitochondria: A target to intrude Alzheimer's disease. Mitochondrion. 2021;**59**:48-57

[140] Fakhri S, Abdian S, Zarneshan SN, Akkol EK, Farzaei MH, Sobarzo-Sánchez E. Targeting mitochondria by plant secondary metabolites: A promising strategy in combating Parkinson's disease. International Journal of Molecular Sciences. 2021;**22**(22):12570

[141] Kita K, Nihei C, Tomitsuka E. Parasite mitochondria as drug target: Diversity and dynamic changes during the life cycle. Current Medicinal Chemistry. 2003;**10**(23):2535-2548

[142] Monzote L, Gille L. Mitochondria as a promising antiparasitic target. Current Clinical Pharmacology. 2010;**5**(1):55-66

[143] Mather M, Henry K, Vaidya A. Mitochondrial drug targets in apicomplexan parasites. Current Drug Targets. 2007;**8**(1):49-60

[144] Sen N, Majumder H. Mitochondrion of protozoan parasite emerges as potent therapeutic target: Exciting drugs are on the horizon. Current Pharmaceutical Design. 2008;**14**(9):839-846

[145] Goodman CD, Buchanan HD, McFadden GI. Is the mitochondrion a good malaria drug target? Trends in Parasitology. 2017;**33**(3):185-193

[146] Nihei C, Fukai Y, Kita K. Trypanosome alternative oxidase as a target of chemotherapy. Biochimica et Biophysica Acta, Molecular Basis of Disease. 2002;**1587**(2-3):234-239

[147] Machado MM. Kinetoplast as a potential chemotherapeutic target of trypanosomatids. Current Pharmaceutical Design. 2008;**14**(9):847-854

[148] Fidalgo LM, Gille L. Mitochondria and trypanosomatids: Targets and drugs. Pharmaceutical Research. 2011;**28**(11):2758-2770

[149] Boveris A, Chance B. The mitochondrial generation of hydrogen

peroxide. General properties and effect of hyperbaric oxygen. The Biochemical Journal. 1973;**134**(3):707-716

[150] Menna-Barreto RFS, de Castro SL. The double-edged sword in pathogenic trypanosomatids: The pivotal role of mitochondria in oxidative stress and bioenergetics. BioMed Research International. 2014;**2014**:1-14

[151] Turrens JF, McCord JM. The iron-containing superoxide dismutases of Trypanosomatidae. Free Radical Biology & Medicine. 2006;**40**(2):193-195

[152] Martínez A, Prolo C, Estrada D, Rios N, Alvarez MN, Piñeyro MD, et al. Cytosolic Fe-superoxide dismutase safeguards *Trypanosoma cruzi* from macrophage-derived superoxide radical. Proceedings of the National Academy of Sciences. 2019;**116**(18):8879-8888

[153] Docampo R, Moreno SN. Free radical metabolism of antiparasitic agents. Federation Proceedings. 1986;**45**(10):2471-2476

[154] Docampo R. Sensitivity of parasites to free radical damage by antiparasitic drugs. Chemico-Biological Interactions. 1990;**73**(1):1-27

[155] Perbandt M, Ndjonka D, Liebau E. Protective mechanisms of Helminths against reactive oxygen species are highly promising drug targets. Current Medicinal Chemistry. 2014;**21**(15):1794-1808

[156] Pal C, Bandyopadhyay U. Redox-active antiparasitic drugs. Antioxidants & Redox Signaling. 2012;**17**(4):555-582

[157] Piacenza L, Irigoín F, Alvarez MN, Peluffo G, Taylor MC, Kelly JM, et al. Mitochondrial superoxide radicals mediate programmed cell death in *Trypanosoma cruzi*: Cytoprotective action of mitochondrial iron superoxide dismutase overexpression. The Biochemical Journal. 2007;**403**(2):323-334

[158] Maya JD, Cassels BK, Iturriaga-Vásquez P, Ferreira J, Faúndez M, Galanti N, et al. Mode of action of natural and synthetic drugs against *Trypanosoma cruzi* and their interaction with the mammalian host. Comparative Biochemistry and Physiology, Part A: Molecular & Integrative Physiology. 2007;**146**(4):601-620

[159] Docampo R, Mason RP, Mottley C, Muniz RP. Generation of free radicals induced by nifurtimox in mammalian tissues. The Journal of Biological Chemistry. 1981;**256**(21):10930-10933

[160] Faúndez M, Rojas M, Bohle P, Reyes C, Letelier ME, Aliaga ME, et al. Pyrogallol red oxidation induced by superoxide radicals: Application to evaluate redox cycling of nitro compounds. Analytical Biochemistry. 2011;**419**(2):284-291

[161] Moreno SNJ, Docampo R, Mason RP, Leon W, Stoppani AOM. Different behaviors of benznidazole as free radical generator with mammalian and *Trypanosoma cruzi* microsomal preparations. Archives of Biochemistry and Biophysics. 1982;**218**(2):585-591

[162] Nogueira FB, Krieger MA, Nirdé P, Goldenberg S, Romanha AJ, Murta SMF. Increased expression of iron-containing superoxide dismutase-A (TcFeSOD-A) enzyme in *Trypanosoma cruzi* population with in vitro-induced resistance to benznidazole. Acta Tropica. 2006;**100**(1-2):119-132

[163] Campos MC, Phelan J, Francisco AF, Taylor MC, Lewis MD, Pain A, et al. Genome-wide mutagenesis and multi-drug resistance in American

trypanosomes induced by the front-line drug benznidazole. Scientific Reports. 2017;**7**(1):14407

[164] Andrade HM, Murta SMF, Chapeaurouge A, Perales J, Nirdé P, Romanha AJ. Proteomic analysis of *Trypanosoma cruzi* resistance to benznidazole. Journal of Proteome Research. 2008;**7**(6):2357-2367

[165] Quebrada Palacio LP, González MN, Hernandez-Vasquez Y, Perrone AE, Parodi-Talice A, Bua J, et al. Phenotypic diversity and drug susceptibility of *Trypanosoma cruzi* TcV clinical isolates. PLoS One. 2018;**13**(9):e0203462

[166] Prathalingham SR, Wilkinson SR, Horn D, Kelly JM. Deletion of the *Trypanosoma brucei* superoxide dismutase gene sodb1 increases sensitivity to nifurtimox and benznidazole. Antimicrobial Agents and Chemotherapy. 2007;**51**(2):755-758

[167] Veronica J, Chandrasekaran S, Dayakar A, Devender M, Prajapati VK, Sundar S, et al. Iron superoxide dismutase contributes to miltefosine resistance in *Leishmania donovani*. The FEBS Journal. 2019;**286**(17):3488-3503

[168] Santi AMM, Silva PA, Santos IFM, Murta SMF. Downregulation of FeSOD-A expression in *Leishmania infantum* alters trivalent antimony and miltefosine susceptibility. Parasites & Vectors. 2021;**14**(1):366

[169] Wassmann C, Hellberg A, Tannich E, Bruchhaus I. Metronidazole resistance in the protozoan parasite *Entamoeba histolytica* is associated with increased expression of iron-containing superoxide dismutase and peroxiredoxin and decreased expression of ferredoxin 1 and flavin reductase. The Journal of Biological Chemistry. 1999;**274**(37):26051-26056

[170] Andrade JM, Murta SMF. Functional analysis of cytosolic tryparedoxin peroxidase in antimony-resistant and -susceptible *Leishmania braziliensis* and *Leishmania infantum* lines. Parasites & Vectors. 2014;**7**(1):406

[171] Olmo F, Urbanová K, Rosales MJ, Martín-Escolano R, Sánchez-Moreno M, Marín C. An in vitro iron superoxide dismutase inhibitor decreases the parasitemia levels of *Trypanosoma cruzi* in BALB/c mouse model during acute phase. International Journal for Parasitology: Drugs and Drug Resistance. 2015;**5**(3):110-116

[172] Singh CK, Chhabra G, Ndiaye MA, Garcia-Peterson LM, Mack NJ, Ahmad N. The role of sirtuins in antioxidant and redox signaling. Antioxidants & Redox Signaling. 2018;**28**(8):643-661

[173] Klein MA, Denu JM. Biological and catalytic functions of sirtuin 6 as targets for small-molecule modulators. The Journal of Biological Chemistry. 2020;**295**(32):11021-11041

[174] Huang J-Y, Hirschey MD, Shimazu T, Ho L, Verdin E. Mitochondrial sirtuins. Biochimica et Biophysica Acta, Proteins and Proteomics. 2010;**1804**(8):1645-1651

[175] Wan X, Garg NJ. Sirtuin control of mitochondrial dysfunction, oxidative stress, and inflammation in Chagas disease models. Frontiers in Cellular and Infection Microbiology. 2021;**11**:693051

[176] Chen Y, Zhang J, Lin Y, Lei Q, Guan K, Zhao S, et al. Tumour suppressor SIRT3 deacetylates and activates manganese superoxide dismutase to scavenge ROS. EMBO Reports. 2011;**12**(6):534-541

[177] dos Santos ML, Santana Nunes V, Gomes AAS, Sousa AC de

CN, Fontes MRM, Schenkman S, et al. Mitochondrial sirtuin TcSir2rp3 affects TcSODA activity and oxidative stress response in *Trypanosoma cruzi*. Frontiers in Cellular and Infection Microbiology. 2021;**11**:773410

[178] Davis CD, Brooks L, Calisi C, Bennett BJ, McElroy DM. Beneficial effect of selenium supplementation during murine infection with *Trypanosoma cruzi*. The Journal of Parasitology. 1998;**84**(6):1274-1277

[179] Gomez RM, Solana ME, Levander OA. Host selenium deficiency increases the severity of chronic inflammatory myopathy in *Trypanosoma cruzi*-inoculated mice. The Journal of Parasitology. 2002;**88**(3):541-547

[180] de Souza AP, de Oliveira GM, Vanderpas J, de Castro SL, Rivera MT, Araújo-Jorge TC. Selenium supplementation at low doses contributes to the decrease in heart damage in experimental *Trypanosoma cruzi* infection. Parasitology Research. 2003;**91**(1):51-54

[181] Holanda MT, Mediano MFF, Hasslocher-Moreno AM, Gonzaga BMS, Carvalho ACC, Ferreira RR, et al. Effects of selenium treatment on cardiac function in Chagas heart disease: Results from the STCC randomized trial. eClinicalMedicine. 2021;**40**:101105

[182] Correa-Oliveira R, Araújo-Jorge TC, Rocha MOC, Rivera MT, Nève J, Moreno AHM, et al. Progressive Chagas' cardiomyopathy is associated with low selenium levels. The American Journal of Tropical Medicine and Hygiene. 2002;**66**(6):706-712

[183] Alcolea V, Pérez-Silanes S. Selenium as an interesting option for the treatment of Chagas disease: A review. European Journal of Medicinal Chemistry. 2020;**206**:112673

[184] Maldonado E, Rojas DA, Urbina F, Solari A. The use of antioxidants as potential co-adjuvants to treat chronic Chagas disease. Antioxidants. 2021;**10**(7):1022

[185] Martín-Escolano R, Etxebeste-Mitxeltorena M, Martín-Escolano J, Plano D, Rosales MJ, Espuelas S, et al. Selenium derivatives as promising therapy for Chagas disease: In vitro and in vivo studies. ACS Infectious Diseases. 2021;7(6):1727-1738

[186] de Freitas MRB, da Costa CMB, Pereira LM, do Prado JC, Sala MA, Abrahão AA. The treatment with selenium increases placental parasitismin pregnant Wistar rats infected with the Y strain of *Trypanosoma cruzi*. Immunobiology. 2018;**223**(10):537-543

[187] Kim SJ, Choi MC, Park JM, Chung AS. Antitumor effects of selenium. International Journal of Molecular Sciences. 2021;**22**(21):11844

[188] Zheng Y, Xie T, Li S, Wang W, Wang Y, Cao Z, et al. Effects of selenium as a dietary source on performance, inflammation, cell damage, and reproduction of livestock induced by heat stress: A review. Frontiers in Immunology. 2022;**12**:820853

[189] Orian L, Flohé L. Selenium-catalyzed reduction of hydroperoxides in chemistry and biology. Antioxidants. 2021;**10**(10):1560

[190] Planer JD, Hulverson MA, Arif JA, Ranade RM, Don R, Buckner FS. Synergy testing of FDA-approved drugs identifies potent drug combinations against *Trypanosoma cruzi*. PLoS Neglected Tropical Diseases. 2014;**8**(7):e2977

[191] Kaiser M, Mäser P, Tadoori LP, Ioset J-R, Brun R. Antiprotozoal activity

profiling of approved drugs: A starting point toward drug repositioning. PLoS One. 2015;**10**(8):e0135556

[192] Lehár J, Krueger AS, Avery W, Heilbut AM, Johansen LM, Price ER, et al. Synergistic drug combinations tend to improve therapeutically relevant selectivity. Nature Biotechnology. 2009;**27**(7):659-666

[193] Lehar J, Krueger AS, Zimmermann GR, Borisy AA. Therapeutic selectivity and the multi-node drug target. Discovery Medicine. 2009;**8**(43):185-190

[194] Zimmermann GR, Lehár J, Keith CT. Multi-target therapeutics: When the whole is greater than the sum of the parts. Drug Discovery Today. 2007;**12**(1-2):34-42

[195] Borisy AA, Elliott PJ, Hurst NW, Lee MS, Lehar J, Price ER, et al. Systematic discovery of multicomponent therapeutics. Proceedings of the National Academy of Sciences. 2003;**100**(13):7977-7982

[196] Kabir A, Muth A. Polypharmacology: The science of multi-targeting molecules. Pharmacological Research. 2022;**176**:106055

[197] Aguilera E, Alvarez G, Cerecetto H, González M. Polypharmacology in the treatment of Chagas disease. Current Medicinal Chemistry. 2019;**26**(23):4476-4489

[198] Mitchison DA. Prevention of drug resistance by combined drug treatment of tuberculosis. In: Coates, A, editor. Antibiotic Resistance. Handbook of Experimental Pharmacology. Springer, Berlin, Heidelberg. 2012;**211**:87-98

[199] Worthington RJ, Melander C. Combination approaches to combat multidrug-resistant bacteria. Trends in Biotechnology. 2013;**31**(3):177-184

[200] Hill JA, Cowen LE. Using combination therapy to thwart drug resistance. Future Microbiology. 2015;**10**(11):1719-1726

[201] Yadav B, Wennerberg K, Aittokallio T, Tang J. Searching for drug synergy in complex dose–response landscapes using an interaction potency model. Computational and Structural Biotechnology Journal. 2015;**13**:504-513

[202] Singh N, Yeh PJ. Suppressive drug combinations and their potential to combat antibiotic resistance. Journal of Antibiotics (Tokyo). 2017;**70**(11):1033-1042

[203] Wani M, Ahmad A. Combination Therapy Against Multidrug Resistance. 1st ed. London: Elsevier, Academic Press; 2020. 260 p

[204] Liu Y, Tong Z, Shi J, Li R, Upton M, Wang Z. Drug repurposing for next-generation combination therapies against multidrug-resistant bacteria. Theranostics. 2021;**11**(10):4910-4928

[205] Wongsrichanalai C, Pickard AL, Wernsdorfer WH, Meshnick SR. Epidemiology of drug-resistant malaria. The Lancet Infectious Diseases. 2002;**2**(4):209-218

[206] Tu Y. From *Artemisia annua* L. to Artemisinins the Discovery and Development of Artemisinins and Antimalarial Agents. 1st ed. London: Agents Academic Press; 2017. 468 p

[207] Ashley EA, Dhorda M, Fairhurst RM, Amaratunga C, Lim P, Suon S, et al. Spread of Artemisinin resistance in *Plasmodium falciparum* malaria. The New England Journal of Medicine. 2014;**371**(5):411-423

[208] Eastman RT, Fidock DA. Artemisinin-based combination

therapies: A vital tool in efforts to eliminate malaria. Nature Reviews. Microbiology. 2009;7(12):864-874

[209] Rogers WO, Sem R, Tero T, Chim P, Lim P, Muth S, et al. Failure of artesunate-mefloquine combination therapy for uncomplicated *Plasmodium falciparum* malaria in Southern Cambodia. Malaria Journal. 2009;**8**(1):10

[210] Lim P, Alker AP, Khim N, Shah NK, Incardona S, Doung S, et al. Pfmdr1 copy number and arteminisin derivatives combination therapy failure in falciparum malaria in Cambodia. Malaria Journal. 2009;**8**(1):11

[211] Alker AP, Lim P, Sem R, Shah NK, Yi P, Bouth DM, et al. Pfmdr1 and in vivo resistance to artesunate-mefloquine in falciparum malaria on the Cambodian-Thai border. The American Journal of Tropical Medicine and Hygiene. 2007;**76**(4):641-647

[212] Nosengo N. Can you teach old drugs new tricks? Nature. 2016;**534**(7607):314-316

[213] Xue H, Li J, Xie H, Wang Y. Review of drug repositioning approaches and resources. International Journal of Biological Sciences. 2018;**14**(10):1232-1244

[214] Simões-Silva MR, De Araújo JS, Peres RB, Da Silva PB, Batista MM, De Azevedo LD, et al. Repurposing strategies for Chagas disease therapy: The effect of imatinib and derivatives against *Trypanosoma cruzi*. Parasitology. 2019;**146**(8):1006-1012

[215] Juárez-Saldivar A, Schroeder M, Salentin S, Haupt VJ, Saavedra E, Vázquez C, et al. Computational drug repositioning for Chagas disease using protein-ligand interaction profiling. International Journal of Molecular Sciences. 2020;**21**(12):4270

[216] Trindade JDS, Freire-de-Lima CG, Côrte-Real S, Decote-Ricardo D, Freire de Lima ME. Drug repurposing for Chagas disease: In vitro assessment of nimesulide against *Trypanosoma cruzi* and insights on its mechanisms of action. PLoS One. 2021;**16**(10):e0258292

[217] Martinez-Peinado N, Cortes-Serra N, Sherman J, Rodriguez A, Bustamante JM, Gascon J, et al. Identification of *Trypanosoma cruzi* growth inhibitors with activity in vivo within a collection of licensed drugs. Microorganisms. 2021;**9**(2):406

[218] Rivero CV, Martínez SJ, Novick P, Cueto JA, Salassa BN, Vanrell MC, et al. Repurposing Carvedilol as a novel inhibitor of the *Trypanosoma cruzi* autophagy flux that affects parasite replication and survival. Frontiers in Cellular and Infection Microbiology. 2021;**11**:657257

[219] Valsecchi WM, Delfino JM, Santos J, Fernández Villamil SH. Zoledronate repositioning as a potential trypanocidal drug. *Trypanosoma cruzi* HPRT an alternative target to be considered. Biochemical Pharmacology. 2021;**188**:114524

[220] Bellera CL, Alberca LN, Sbaraglini ML, Talevi A. In silico drug repositioning for Chagas disease. Current Medicinal Chemistry. 2020;**27**(5):662-675

[221] Reigada C, Sayé M, Phanstiel O, Valera-Vera E, Miranda MR, Pereira CA. Identification of *Trypanosoma cruzi* polyamine transport inhibitors by computational drug repurposing. Frontiers in Medicine. 2019;**6**:256

[222] Valera-Vera EA, Sayé M, Reigada C, Miranda MR, Pereira CA. In

silico repositioning of etidronate as a potential inhibitor of the *Trypanosoma cruzi* enolase. Journal of Molecular Graphics & Modelling. 2020;**95**: 107506

[223] Miranda MR, Sayé MM. Chagas disease treatment: From new therapeutic targets to drug discovery and repositioning. Current Medicinal Chemistry. 2019;**26**(36):6517-6518

[224] Santos SS, de Araújo RV, Giarolla J, Seoud O El, Ferreira EI. Searching for drugs for Chagas disease, leishmaniasis and schistosomiasis: A review. International Journal of Antimicrobial Agents 2020;55(4):105906.

[225] Adasme MF, Bolz SN, Adelmann L, Salentin S, Haupt VJ, Moreno-Rodríguez A, et al. Repositioned drugs for Chagas disease unveiled via structure-based drug repositioning. International Journal of Molecular Sciences. 2020;**21**(22):8809

[226] Martínez-Flórez A, Galizzi M, Izquierdo L, Bustamante JM, Rodriguez A, Rodriguez F, et al. Repurposing bioenergetic modulators against protozoan parasites responsible for tropical diseases. International Journal for Parasitology: Drugs and Drug Resistance. 2020;**14**:17-27

[227] Benaim G, Paniz-Mondolfi AE, Sordillo EM. The rationale for use of amiodarone and its derivatives for the treatment of Chagas' disease and Leishmaniasis. Current Pharmaceutical Design. 2021;**27**(15):1825-1833

[228] Zuma AA, de Souza W. Chagas disease chemotherapy: What do we know so far? Current Pharmaceutical Design. 2021;**27**(38):3963-3995

[229] Torrico F, Gascón J, Barreira F, Blum B, Almeida IC, Alonso-Vega C, et al. New regimens of benznidazole monotherapy and in combination with fosravuconazole for treatment of Chagas disease (BENDITA): A phase 2, double-blind, randomised trial. The Lancet Infectious Diseases. 2021;**21**(8):1129-1140

[230] Mazzeti AL, Gonçalves KR, Mota SLA, Pereira DE, Diniz L, Bahia MT. Combination therapy using nitro compounds improves the efficacy of experimental Chagas disease treatment. Parasitology. 2021;**148**(11):1320-1327

[231] Mazzeti AL, Capelari-Oliveira P, Bahia MT, Mosqueira VCF. Review on experimental treatment strategies against *Trypanosoma cruzi*. Journal of Experimental Pharmacology. 2021;**13**:409-432

[232] Peerzada MN, Gaur A, Azam A. Advances in drug discovery against neglected tropical diseases: Human African and American Trypanosomiasis. Current Medicinal Chemistry. 2021;**28**(36):7544-7582

[233] Ferraz LRM, Silva LC, de Souza ML, Alves LP, de Sales V, Barbosa NG, et al. Drug associations as alternative and complementary therapy for neglected tropical diseases. Acta Tropica. 2022;**225**:106210

[234] Araujo-Lima CF, Peres RB, Silva PB, Batista MM, Aiub CAF, Felzenszwalb I, et al. Repurposing strategy of atorvastatin against *Trypanosoma cruzi*: In vitro monotherapy and combined therapy with benznidazole exhibit synergistic trypanocidal activity. Antimicrobial Agents and Chemotherapy. 2018;**62**(9):e00979-18

[235] Sass G, Madigan RT, Joubert L-M, Bozzi A, Sayed N, Wu JC, et al. A combination of itraconazole and amiodarone is highly effective against

*Trypanosoma cruzi* infection of human stem cell-derived cardiomyocytes. The American Journal of Tropical Medicine and Hygiene. 2019;**101**(2):383-391

[236] Simões-Silva MR, De Araújo JS, Oliveira GM, Demarque KC, Peres RB, D'Almeida-Melo I, et al. Drug repurposing strategy against *Trypanosoma cruzi* infection: In vitro and in vivo assessment of the activity of metronidazole in mono- and combined therapy. Biochemical Pharmacology. 2017;**145**:46-53

[237] Sun W, Sanderson PE, Zheng W. Drug combination therapy increases successful drug repositioning. Drug Discovery Today. 2016;**21**(7):1189-1195

[238] Pandey RP, Nascimento MS, Moore CE, Raj VS, Kalil J, Cunha-Neto E. New approaches for the treatment of Chagas disease. Current Drug Targets. 2021;**22**(7):835-841

[239] Sousa A. Disulfiram: Its Use in Alcohol Dependence and Other Disorders. 1st ed. Singapore: Springer; 2019. 133 p

[240] Suh JJ, Pettinati HM, Kampman KM, O'Brien CP. The status of disulfiram. Journal of Clinical Psychopharmacology. 2006;**26**(3):290-302

[241] Bala V, Gupta G, Sharma V. Chemical and medicinal versatility of dithiocarbamates: An overview. Mini Reviews in Medicinal Chemistry. 2014;**14**(12):1021-1032

[242] Shinde SD, Sakla AP, Shankaraiah N. An insight into medicinal attributes of dithiocarbamates: Bird's eye view. Bioorganic Chemistry. 2020;**105**:104346

[243] Gessner PK, Gessner T. Disulfiram and Its Metabolite, Diethyldithiocarbamate. Dordrecht: Springer Netherlands; 1992

[244] Rath NC, Rasaputra KS, Liyanage R, Huff GR and Huff WE. Dithiocarbamate Toxicity - An Appraisal. In: Stoytcheva M, editor. Pesticides in the Modern World - Effects of Pesticides Exposure. London, UK: InTechOpen; 2011. pp. 323-340

[245] Hald J, Jacobsen E. A drug sensitising the organism to ethyl alcohol. Lancet. 1948;**252**(6539):1001-1004

[246] Lu C, Li X, Ren Y, Zhang X. Disulfiram: A novel repurposed drug for cancer therapy. Cancer Chemotherapy and Pharmacology. 2021;**87**(2):159-172

[247] Jia Y, Huang T. Overview of Antabuse® (Disulfiram) in radiation and cancer biology. Cancer Management and Research. 2021;**13**:4095-4101

[248] Meraz-Torres F, Plöger S, Garbe C, Niessner H, Sinnberg T. Disulfiram as a therapeutic agent for metastatic malignant melanoma—Old myth or new logos? Cancers (Basel). 2020;**12**(12):3538

[249] Jiao Y, Hannafon BN, Ding W-Q. Disulfiram's anticancer activity: Evidence and mechanisms. Anti-Cancer Agents in Medicinal Chemistry. 2016;**16**(11):1378-1384

[250] Spivak AM, Planelles V. Novel latency reversal agents for HIV-1 cure. Annual Review of Medicine. 2018;**69**(1):421-436

[251] de Moura FB, Kohut SJ, Bergman J. Limited modulation of the abuse-related behavioral effects of d-methamphetamine by disulfiram. Experimental and Clinical Psychopharmacology. 2018;**26**(5):497-502

[252] Reinhardt S, Stoye N, Luderer M, Kiefer F, Schmitt U, Lieb K, et al. Identification of disulfiram as a secretase-modulating compound with beneficial effects on Alzheimer's

disease hallmarks. Scientific Reports. 2018;**8**(1):1329

[253] Gao J, Gong Z, Montesano D, Glazer E, Liegner K. "Repurposing" disulfiram in the treatment of lyme disease and babesiosis: Retrospective review of first 3 years' experience in one medical practice. Antibiotics. 2020;**9**(12):868

[254] Zitko J, Doležal M. Old drugs and new targets as an outlook for the treatment of tuberculosis. Current Medicinal Chemistry. 2019;**25**(38):5142-5167

[255] Das S, Garg T, Chopra S, Dasgupta A. Repurposing disulfiram to target infections caused by non-tuberculous mycobacteria. The Journal of Antimicrobial Chemotherapy. 2019;**74**(5):1317-1322

[256] Castillo-Villanueva A, Rufino-González Y, Méndez S-T, Torres-Arroyo A, Ponce-Macotela M, Martínez-Gordillo MN, et al. Disulfiram as a novel inactivator of *Giardia lamblia* triosephosphate isomerase with antigiardial potential. International Journal for Parasitology: Drugs and Drug Resistance. 2017;**7**(3):425-432

[257] Shirley D-A, Sharma I, Warren CA, Moonah S. Drug repurposing of the alcohol abuse medication disulfiram as an anti-parasitic agent. Frontiers in Cellular and Infection Microbiology. 2021;**11**:633194

[258] Omran Z, Sheikh R, Baothman OA, Zamzami MA, Alarjah M. Repurposing disulfiram as an anti-obesity drug: Treating and preventing obesity in high-fat-fed rats. Diabetes, Metabolic Syndrome and Obesity: Targets and Therapy. 2020;**13**:1473-1480

[259] Kannappan V, Ali M, Small B, Rajendran G, Elzhenni S, Taj H, et al. Recent advances in repurposing disulfiram and disulfiram derivatives as copper-dependent anticancer agents. Frontiers in Molecular Biosciences. 2021;**8**:741316

[260] Fong W, To KK. Drug repurposing to overcome resistance to various therapies for colorectal cancer. Cellular and Molecular Life Sciences. 2019;**76**(17):3383-3406

[261] Ekinci E, Rohondia S, Khan R, Dou QP. Repurposing disulfiram as an anti-cancer agent: Updated review on literature and patents. Recent Patents on Anti-Cancer Drug Discovery. 2019;**14**(2):113-132

[262] Horita Y, Takii T, Yagi T, Ogawa K, Fujiwara N, Inagaki E, et al. Antitubercular activity of disulfiram, an antialcoholism drug, against multidrug- and extensively drug-resistant mycobacterium tuberculosis isolates. Antimicrobial Agents and Chemotherapy. 2012;**56**(8):4140-4145

[263] Long TE. Repurposing thiram and disulfiram as antibacterial agents for *multidrug-resistant Staphylococcus aureus* infections. Antimicrobial Agents and Chemotherapy. 2017;**61**(9):e00898-17

[264] Sauna ZE, Shukla S, Ambudkar SV. Disulfiram, an old drug with new potential therapeutic uses for human cancers and fungal infections. Molecular BioSystems. 2005;**1**(2):127

[265] Argüello-García R, Leitsch D, Skinner-Adams T, Ortega-Pierres MG. Drug resistance in Giardia: Mechanisms and alternative treatments for Giardiasis. Advances in Parasitology. 2020;**107**:201-282

[266] Cvek B. Nonprofit drugs as the salvation of the world's healthcare

systems: The case of Antabuse (disulfiram). Drug Discovery Today. 2012;**17**(9-10):409-412

[267] Jørgensen CH, Pedersen B, Tønnesen H. The efficacy of disulfiram for the treatment of alcohol use disorder. Alcoholism, Clinical and Experimental Research. 2011;**35**(10):1749-1758

[268] Sinclair JMA, Chambers SE, Shiles CJ, Baldwin DS. Safety and tolerability of pharmacological treatment of alcohol dependence: Comprehensive review of evidence. Drug Safety. 2016;**39**(7):627-645

[269] Reisinger EC, Kern P, Dietrich M, Ernst M, Flad HD, Bock P, et al. Inhibition of HIV progression by dithiocarb. Lancet. 1990;**335**(8691):679-682

[270] Pompidou A, Delsaux MC, Telvi L, Mace B, Coutance F, Falkenrodt A, et al. Isoprinosine and Imuthiol, two potentially active compounds in patients with AIDS-related complex symptoms. Cancer Research. 1985;**45**(9):4671-4673

[271] Lemarie E, Musset M, Charbonnier C, Renoux M, Renoux G. Clinical characterization of imuthiol. Methods and Findings in Experimental and Clinical Pharmacology. 1986;**8**(1):51-54

[272] Khouri R, Novais F, Santana G, de Oliveira CI, Vannier dos Santos MA, Barral A, et al. DETC induces leishmania parasite killing in human in vitro and murine in vivo models: A promising therapeutic alternative in leishmaniasis. PLoS One. 2010;**5**(12):e14394

[273] Assolini JP, Tomiotto-Pellissier F, da Silva Bortoleti BT, Gonçalves MD, Sahd CS, Carloto ACM, et al. Diethyldithiocarbamate encapsulation reduces toxicity and promotes leishmanicidal effect through apoptosis-like mechanism in promastigote and ROS production by macrophage. Journal of Drug Targeting. 2020;**28**(10):1110-1123

[274] Mazur KL, Feuser PE, Valério A, Poester Cordeiro A, de Oliveira CI, Assolini JP, et al. Diethyldithiocarbamate loaded in beeswax-copaiba oil nanoparticles obtained by solventless double emulsion technique promote promastigote death in vitro. Colloids and Surfaces. B, Biointerfaces. 2019;**176**:507-512

[275] Celes FS, Trovatti E, Khouri R, Van Weyenbergh J, Ribeiro SJL, Borges VM, et al. DETC-based bacterial cellulose bio-curatives for topical treatment of cutaneous leishmaniasis. Scientific Reports. 2016;**6**(1):38330

[276] McMahon A, Chen W, Li F. Old wine in new bottles: Advanced drug delivery systems for disulfiram-based cancer therapy. Journal of Controlled Release. 2020;**319**:352-359

[277] Kyle ME, Serroni A, Farber JL. The inhibition of lipid peroxidation by disulfiram prevents the killing of cultured hepatocytes by allyl alcohol, tert-butyl hydroperoxide, hydrogen peroxide and diethyl maleate. Chemico-Biological Interactions. 1989;**72**(3):269-275

[278] Liu T, Wang P, Cong M, Zhao X, Zhang D, Xu H, et al. Diethyldithiocarbamate, an anti-abuse drug, alleviates steatohepatitis and fibrosis in rodents through modulating lipid metabolism and oxidative stress. British Journal of Pharmacology. 2018;**175**(24):4480-4495

[279] Sundar S, Chakravarty J, Meena LP. Leishmaniasis: Treatment, drug resistance and emerging therapies.

Expert Opinion on Orphan Drugs. 2019;7(1):1-10

[280] Calle LM, Sullivan PD. Screening of antioxidants and other compounds for antimutagenic properties towards benzo[a]pyrene-induced mutagenicity in strain TA98 of *Salmonella typhimurium*. Mutation Research. 1982;**101**(2):99-114

[281] Lane JE, Ribeiro-Rodrigues R, Suarez CC, Bogitsh BJ, Jones MM, Singh PK, et al. In vitro trypanocidal activity of tetraethylthiuram disulfide and sodium diethylamine-N-carbodithioate on *Trypanosoma cruzi*. The American Journal of Tropical Medicine and Hygiene. 1996;**55**(3):263-266

[282] de Freitas Oliveira JW, Torres TM, Moreno CJG, Amorim-Carmo B, Damasceno IZ, Soares AKMC, et al. Insights of antiparasitic activity of sodium diethyldithiocarbamate against different strains of *Trypanosoma cruzi*. Scientific Reports. 2021;**11**(1):11200

[283] Giulivi C, Turrens JF, Boveris A. Chemiluminescence enhancement by trypanocidal drugs and by inhibitors of antioxidant enzymes in *Trypanosoma cruzi*. Molecular and Biochemical Parasitology. 1988;**30**(3):243-251

[284] Koto KS, Lescault P, Brard L, Kim K, Singh RK, Bond J, et al. Antitumor activity of nifurtimox is enhanced with tetrathiomolybdate in medulloblastoma. International Journal of Oncology. 2011;**38**(5):1329-1341

[285] Prentice H, Modi JP, Wu J-Y. Mechanisms of neuronal protection against excitotoxicity, endoplasmic reticulum stress, and mitochondrial dysfunction in stroke and neurodegenerative diseases. Oxidative Medicine and Cellular Longevity. 2015;**2015**:1-7

[286] Masuda Y, Nakayama N. Protective action of diethyldithiocarbamate and carbon disulfide against renal injury induced by chloroform in mice. Biochemical Pharmacology. 1983;**32**(21):3127-3135

[287] Gandhi NM, Gopalaswamy UV, Nair CKK. Radiation protection by disulfiram: Protection of membrane and DNA in vitro and in vivo against γ-radiation. Journal of Radiation Research. 2003;**44**(3):255-259

[288] Gandhi NM, Nair CKK. Radiation protection by diethyldithiocarbamate: Protection of membrane and DNA in vitro and in vivo against γ-radiation. Journal of Radiation Research. 2004;**45**(2):175-180

[289] Wysor MS, Zwelling LA, Sanders JE, Grenan MM. Cure of mice infected with *Trypanosoma rhodesiense* by cis-diamminedichloroplatinum (ii) and disulfiram rescue. Science 80. 1982;**217**(4558):454-456

[290] Ishikawa M, Aoki T, Yomogida S, Takayanagi Y, Sasaki K. Drug interaction effects on antitumour drugs (XV): Disulfiram as protective agent against cyclophosphamide-induced urotoxicity without compromising antitumour activity in mice. Pharmacology & Toxicology. 1994;**74**(6):255-261

[291] Ishikawa M, Takayanagi Y, Sasaki K. Inhibition of ifosfamide-induced urotoxicity by disulfiram in mice. Japanese Journal of Pharmacology. 1989;**49**(1):147-150

[292] Brambilla G, Carlo P, Finollo R. Effect of ten thiocompounds on rat liver DNA damage induced by a small dose of N-nitrosodimethylamine. Archives of Toxicology. 1992;**66**(4):286-290

[293] Burman WJ, Terra M, Breese P, Cohn D, Reves R. Lack of toxicity from concomitant directly observed disulfiram and isoniazid-containing therapy for active tuberculosis. The International Journal of Tuberculosis and Lung Disease. 2002;**6**(9):839-842

[294] Traiger GJ, Vyas KP, Hanzlik RP. Effect of thiocarbonyl compounds on α-naphthylisothiocyanate-induced hepatotoxicity and the urinary excretion of [35S]α-naphthylisothiocyanate in the rat. Toxicology and Applied Pharmacology. 1984;**72**(3):504-512

[295] Hazai E, Vereczkey L, Monostory K. Reduction of toxic metabolite formation of acetaminophen. Biochemical and Biophysical Research Communications. 2002;**291**(4):1089-1094

[296] Kim HL, Jones LP. Protective effects of butylated hydroxyanisole, ethoxyquin, and disulfiram on acute pyrrolizidine alkaloids poisoning in mice. Research Communications in Chemical Pathology and Pharmacology. 1982;**36**(2):341-344

[297] Masukawa T, Nakanishi K. Protection by disulfiram and diethyldithiocarbamate against hypoxia-induced lethality in mice. Japanese Journal of Pharmacology. 1993;**63**(3):279-284

[298] Jennische E, Hansson H. Disulfiram is protective against postischemic cell death in the liver. Acta Physiologica Scandinavica. 1984;**122**(2):199-201

[299] Llobet JM, Domingo JL, Paternain JL, Corbella J. Treatment of acute lead intoxication. A quantitative comparison of a number of chelating agents. Archives of Environmental Contamination and Toxicology. 1990;**19**(2):185-189

[300] Hiroshige Ono Takayuki Funakoshi H. Comparative effects of disulfiram and diethyldithiocarbamate against testicular toxicity in rats caused by acute exposure to cadmium. Journal of Toxicology and Environmental Health. 1997;**50**(4):389-400

[301] Pages A, Casaş JS, Sanchez A, Sordo J, Bravo J, Gayoso M. Dithiocarbamates in heavy metal poisoning: Complexes of N,N-di(2-hidroxyethyl)dithiocarbamate with Zn(II), Cd(II), Hg(II), CH3Hg(II), and C6H5Hg(II). Journal of Inorganic Biochemistry. 1985;**25**(1):35-42

[302] Cohen G, Heikkila RE, Allis B, Cabbat F, Dembiec D, MacNamee D, et al. Destruction of sympathetic nerve terminals by 6-hydroxydopamine: Protection by 1-phenyl-3-(2-thiazolyl)-2-thiourea, diethyldithiocarbamate, methimazole, cysteamine, ethanol and n-butanol. The Journal of Pharmacology and Experimental Therapeutics. 1976;**199**(2):336-352

[303] Sonawane VK, Mahajan UB, Shinde SD, Chatterjee S, Chaudhari SS, Bhangale HA, et al. A chemosensitizer drug: Disulfiram prevents doxorubicin-induced cardiac dysfunction and oxidative stress in rats. Cardiovascular Toxicology. 2018;**18**(5):459-470

[304] Kis A, Yellon DM, Baxter GF. Role of nuclear factor-κB activation in acute ischaemia-reperfusion injury in myocardium. British Journal of Pharmacology. 2003;**138**(5):894-900

[305] McPherson BC, Yao Z. Signal transduction of opioid-induced cardioprotection in ischemia-reperfusion. Anesthesiology. 2001;**94**(6):1082-1088

[306] Wei S, Xiao Z, Huang J, Peng Z, Zhang B, Li W. Disulfiram

inhibits oxidative stress and NLRP3 inflammasome activation to prevent LPS-induced cardiac injury. International Immunopharmacology. 2022;**105**:108545

[307] Köksoy FN, Köse H, Soybír GR, Yalçin O, Cokneşelí B. The prophylactic effects of superoxide dismutase, catalase, desferrioxamine, verapamil and disulfiram in experimental colitis. Journal of the Royal College of Surgeons of Edinburgh. 1997;**42**(1):27-30

[308] Campos MCO, Castro-Pinto DB, Ribeiro GA, Berredo-Pinho MM, Gomes LHF, da Silva Bellieny MS, et al. P-glycoprotein efflux pump plays an important role in *Trypanosoma cruzi* drug resistance. Parasitology Research. 2013;**112**(6):2341-2351

[309] Loo TW, Bartlett MC, Clarke DM. Disulfiram metabolites permanently inactivate the human multidrug resistance P-glycoprotein. Molecular Pharmaceutics. 2004;**1**(6):426-433

[310] Sauna ZE, Peng X-H, Nandigama K, Tekle S, Ambudkar SV. The molecular basis of the action of disulfiram as a modulator of the multidrug resistance-linked ATP binding cassette transporters MDR1 (ABCB1) and MRP1 (ABCC1). Molecular Pharmacology. 2004;**65**(3):675-684

[311] da Costa KM, Valente RC, Salustiano EJ, Gentile LB, Freire-de-Lima L, Mendonça-Previato L, et al. Functional characterization of ABCC proteins from *Trypanosoma cruzi* and their involvement with thiol transport. Frontiers in Microbiology. 2018;**9**:205

[312] Jin L, Davis MR, Hu P, Baillie TA. Identification of novel glutathione conjugates of disulfiram and diethyldithiocarbamate in rat bile by liquid chromatography-tandem mass spectrometry. Evidence for metabolic activation of disulfiram in vivo. Chemical Research in Toxicology. 1994;**7**(4):526-533

[313] Giustarini D, Galvagni F, Tesei A, Farolfi A, Zanoni M, Pignatta S, et al. Glutathione, glutathione disulfide, and S-glutathionylated proteins in cell cultures. Free Radical Biology & Medicine. 2015;**89**:972-981

[314] Arnelle DR, Day BJ, Stamler JS. Diethyl dithiocarbamate-induced decomposition of S-Nitrosothiols. Nitric Oxide. 1997;**1**(1):56-64

[315] Johnston CD. The in vitro reaction between tetraethylthiuram disulfide (antabuse) and glutathione. Archives of Biochemistry and Biophysics. 1953;**44**(1):249-251

[316] Goldstein BD, Rozen MG, Quintavalla JC, Amoruso MA. Decrease in mouse lung and liver glutathione peroxidase activity and potentiation of the lethal effects of ozone and paraquat by the superoxide dismutase inhibitor diethyldithio-carbamate. Biochemical Pharmacology. 1979;**28**(1):27-30

[317] Kona R, Buac D, Burger M. Disulfiram, and disulfiram derivatives as novel potential anticancer drugs targeting the ubiquitin proteasome system in both preclinical and clinical studies. Current Cancer Drug Targets. 2011;**11**(3):338-346

[318] Gupta I, Aggarwal S, Singh K, Yadav A, Khan S. Ubiquitin proteasome pathway proteins as potential drug targets in parasite *Trypanosoma cruzi*. Scientific Reports. 2018;**8**(1):8399

[319] Banerjee ER. Perspectives in Translational Research in Life Sciences and Biomedicine. Springer Singapore: Singapore; 2016

[320] Saraiva RM, Portela LF, Silveira GPE da, da Gomes NL, Pinto DP, de Silva AC, et al. Disulfiram repurposing in the combined chemotherapy of Chagas disease. Medicine: Case Reports and Study Protocols. 2021;**2**(7):e0110

Section 3

# The Pathogenesis

Chapter 5

# Digestive Disorders in Chagas Disease: Megaesophagus and Chagasic Megacolon

*Víctor Hugo García Orozco, Juan Enrique Villalvazo Navarro, Carlos Solar Aguirre, Carlos Manuel Ibarra Ocampo, César Iván Díaz Sandoval, Carlos Alejandro Ortíz Gallegos, Diego Javier Oregel Camacho and Araceli Noriega Bucio*

## Abstract

Chagas disease, also known as American trypanosomiasis, caused by *Trypanosoma cruzi* and transmitted by hematophagous vectors, is a parasitic disease, which according to the WHO ranks fourth as a cause of loss of potential years of life due to complications that can occur in multiple body systems. According to the reports presented by the World Health Organization, there are between 16 and 18 million infected people in the world, predominantly in endemic areas of Latin America, of which only 1% receives an adequate diagnosis and full treatment, thereby that the chronic phase comes to present digestive disorders that are one of the main causes of loss in the quality of life of patients, as well as complications that can lead to life-threatening surgical emergencies.

**Keywords:** Chagas disease, megacolon, megaesophagus, trypanosomiasis, digestive disorders, achalasia, occlusion

## 1. Introduction

American trypanosomiasis ranks as the fourth most frequent disease-causing loss of productive years [1]. Also known as Chagas disease, this disease is a parasitic infection transmitted by hematophagous vectors [2] and is characterized by an acute period with general symptoms, which leads to a chronic phase and the development of complications at different levels of the infected organism. The reports, made by the World Health Organization (WHO), mention that in the world there are between 16 and 18 million infected people which approximately only 1% receives an early diagnosis and full treatment, being the area with the highest incidence is in the Latin American area where this infection is considered endemic. Due to the public health implications and the high percentage of complications that it presents in chronic phases, the Pan-American organization and the World Health Organization consider this disease as the most serious parasitic infection in Latin America [1].



IntechOpen

In addition to vector transmission, this infection can be spread vertically through infected women during pregnancy, leading to gestational disease with implications for uterine or neonatal development.

Among the major complications of the chronic stage of Chagas disease, it is the development of the so-called—mega syndromes, within which megaesophagus and Chagasic megacolon are more frequently included, which develop from alterations in the neurosensory system in the muscular layers of these organs. Both scenarios present significant complication rates that condition the loss of productive years, a decrease in the quality of life, and compromise life depending on the presentation of volvulations or eating disorders.

Although the development of complications associated with the chronic stages of Chagas diseases, such as intestinal volvulations [3] in megacolon, is relatively uncommon in Western countries, it is still considered the most severe complication [4], positioning itself as the third cause of lower intestinal obstruction in some countries, only below diverticular disease and colon cancer [1]; with respect to megaesophagus, complications can occur even in patients who are considered asymptomatic, who nevertheless present motor disorders of the esophagus that can lead to the development of neoplasms.

## 2. Background

Chagas disease was discovered in 1909 by Dr. Carlos Chagas, he studied blood-sucking insects with a nocturnal habit called "barbeiros" (**Figure 1**). Chagas sent samples of

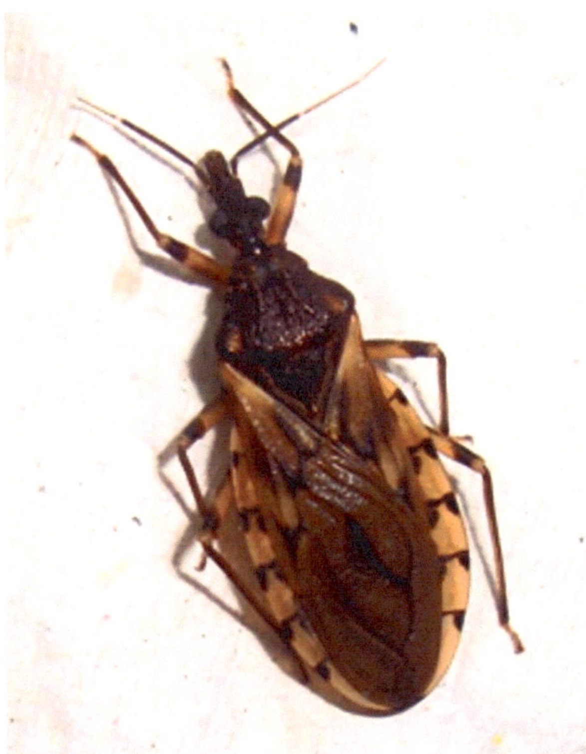

**Figure 1.**
*Hematophagous barbeiro insect causing transmission of Chagas disease.*

Barbeiros that Dr. Cruz inoculated into monkeys. After 30 days, Chagas examined the monkeys' blood and found parasites, which he named *Trypanosoma cruzi*. Together with their colleagues, from 1909 to 1917, they defined the clinical aspects of the disease. The first case described in humans was Berenice, a 2-year-old girl who presented 39.4°C, eyelid edema, adenomegaly, hepatomegaly, and the presence of *T. cruzi* in peripheral blood, with subsequent remission of signs and symptoms [5].

In a study by Aufderheide et al. with the review of mummies exhumed from archeological sites in both Peru and Chile, a carbon dating of their tissues was revealed to approximately 7000 BC. and confirmed by means of the polymerase chain reaction (PCR) the presence of DNA of the *T. cruzi* kinetoplast. Another historical fact dates back to 1835, when Charles Darwin was in Argentina, in the province of Luján de Cuyo in the southern district of Mendoza, he was inoculated by a triatomine insect. He studied these insects for at least 4 months. From 1835 to 1841, Darwin reported no symptoms, which could be due to the latent phase of Chagas disease. From 1841 to 1861, Darwin reported palpitations, a feeling of extreme fatigue, tremors, flatulence, and vomiting to his colleagues and doctors, however, none could identify the cause. At the age of 33, he left his job due to physical fatigue and digestive disorders, which can be explained by Chagas disease, Darwin experienced anginal attacks and was eventually diagnosed with heart failure. Darwin's disease has caused extensive speculation in the scientific community. Two things are clear—1) he was exposed to the triatomine insect and 2) his symptoms can be explained by Chagas disease [6].

## 3. Epidemiological aspects

*T. cruzi* gets its entry into the body through its vector, the triatomines, members of the reduvius family when the insect ingests blood from an infected animal. The protozoan replicates in the intestine of the triatomine and is excreted from its feces. The main route of transmission in humans is the inoculation of feces directly on the mucous membranes, or in skin lesions that are generated by scratching or damage caused by the insect bites. It can also occur by blood transfusion or tissue transplantation (organ or bone marrow) from an infected person and by transmission from the mother to her fetus during pregnancy. There is another way of transmission, the oral route, which occurs when the ingestion of feces from triatomine infected with *T. cruzi*, when the consumption of meat or blood of wild animals, or contamination from utensils for prepare food. The estimated incidence has dropped from 500,000 in 1991 to 30,000 new cases of infection per year in 2010. The annual cost to an individual's society for chronic disease care was $ 4059 (range $ 3569–4434) in Latin America, 13,580 ($ 11,340–15,003) in Europe, and $ 15,762 ($ 13,249–17,442) in the US, Canada and Australia, globally the weighted measure of the annual cost of health care and the productivity of a person with chronic disease was $ 4660, the estimated annual global burden of the disease is $ 627.46 million in health spending and 806,170 disability-adjusted life years, 10% of this burden affects non-endemic countries [7].

In the case of Latin America, 20% of its population is at risk of acquiring the infection, especially in endemic areas. In Mexico, it is considered a public health problem, since it is estimated that 1.1 million people are infected. The incidence from 2000 to 2007 remained in the range of 0.07–0.37 per 100,000 people, increasing to 0.70 in 2012. During 2018, 150 cases were registered throughout the republic. According to a 2013–2018 report, Chagas disease is the most serious parasitic disease in Latin

America, since there are 110 million people at risk of infection in 21 different countries, likewise, the World Health Organization has classified it as one of the 14 lagging diseases [8].

## 4. Pathophysiology

The *T. cruzi* parasite is a heterogeneous species with a diverse phenotypic diversity, circulates between vectors and hosts, and is classified into discrete typing units a term used to describe sets of stocks that are genetically similar to each other and have "tags" a molecular marker to identify each other DTU (TcI-TcIVI and Tcbat) [9]. The life cycle consists of three different forms, metacyclic trypomastigotes, the infection form of *T. cruzi*, which consists of a fusiform shape and measures 10–20 m in length and 1.3 m in width. The transmitted by feces while triatomines feed on blood they defecate on the skin and *T. cruzi* introduces itself through the opening made by the bite and enter to the bloodstream or by rubbing on the mucosae (nasal or conjunctival). In the body, they are phagocytosed by macrophages, in the cytosol of subcutaneous cellular tissue they differentiate into amastigotes. The amastigotes measure 1.5–5 m in diameter with an ovoid shape, they replicate by binary fission and cause cell lysis to turn back to trypomastigotes to go into the blood and lymphatic circulation, they have tropism for myocardiocytes, rhabdomyocytes, and leiomyocytes. In this phase, a vector without infection can ingest it, within triatomines, trypomastigotes move to the medial segment of the gastrointestinal tract, once there they differentiate into epimastigotes, which replicate again through binary fission. Epimastigotes travel toward the distal segment of the gastrointestinal tract where they anchor themselves to colon epithelium through their flagella, they transform back to trypomastigotes to be excreted with feces during the next ingestion of blood and infect another human [8, 10]. In addition to vector transmission, *T. cruzi* can be transmitted by routes other than direct inoculation. These transmission routes play a greater role in non-endemic countries and a significant growth in endemic areas. It is estimated that vertical transmission reaches a frequency of 4.7% (range 3.9–5.6%) and that frequency may be higher in endemic countries than in non-endemic countries (5 vs. 2.7%). The biological determinant for congenital transmission is maternal parasitemia, which can be greater than 31% when *T. cruzi* is detected by PCR, likewise, transmission is also possible although it presents negative PCR [11]. The parasite can also be transmitted through blood and its products, the frequency of transmission per unit of infected blood is estimated to be 10–25%. In solid organ transplants from an infected donor, it appears to be lower for kidney recipients (0–19%) than for liver recipients (0–29%) and heart recipients (75–100%) [11].

The acute phase of Chagas disease is characterized by strong inhibition of the host's immune response triggered by virulence factors of *T. cruzi*, which are crucial to create a persistent infection and establish chronic disease involving, among other things, the induction of anergy and clonal deletion in T cell compartments, together with strong polyclonal stimulation of type B cells which restrict antigen-specific lymphocytes. Membrane glycoproteins of *T. cruzi* are essential to dampen the host's protective immunity. These membranes are covered by mucin-like molecules attached to their terminal galactosyl residues, sialic acid residues that are transferred from host glycoconjugates by parasite trans-sialidase. Mucin-like molecules of *T. cruzi* are key players in host–parasite interaction, including invasion of the host and subversion of its immune system. Its sialylated forms are capable of protecting the antigenic determinants of the parasite from host attack mediated by antigalactosyl antibodies and complement factor B. Likewise, they incapacitate dendritic cell function demonstrated by the inhibition of IL-12 production. This inhibition can occur at the transcriptional level of the IL-2 gene in T cells, which also occurs when T cell proliferation and activation are blocked in response to mitogens and antigens. Sialoglycoproteins also inhibit early events in T cell activation, particularly tyrosine phosphorylation of the adapter protein SLP-76 and tyrosine kinase ZAP-70 [12].

## 5. Clinical presentation

As mentioned above, Chagas disease has two phases of development, the acute and the chronic period. The acute phase can occur at any age, has an incubation period of 4–14 days, and a duration of 2–4 months. It is asymptomatic in 95% of cases when symptoms occur, these include fever (75%), inflammation in the inoculation site (inoculation chagoma, 25%), unilateral eyelid edema (Romaña-Mazza sign; when the conjunctiva is the gateway, 50%) (**Figure 2**), lymphadenopathy, and hepatosplenomegaly. The acute phase lasts 4–8 weeks, and parasitemia decreases substantially from day 90 onwards. A severe acute phase occurs in less than 1–5% of patients, including manifestations, such as acute myocarditis, pleural effusion, and meningoencephalitis (mortality risk 0.2–0.5% [8].

Cases of congenital infection are generally characterized by the absence of symptoms in 70–80% of cases. The remaining 20–30% may have signs and symptoms, such as prematurity, low weight for gestational age, edema, jaundice, respiratory distress, persistent tachycardia, hepatosplenomegaly, and anemia. Occasionally sepsis, fever, hydrops fetalis, rash, petechiae, lymphadenopathy, meningoencephalitis, cerebral calcifications, fundus abnormalities, interstitial pneumonia, myocarditis.

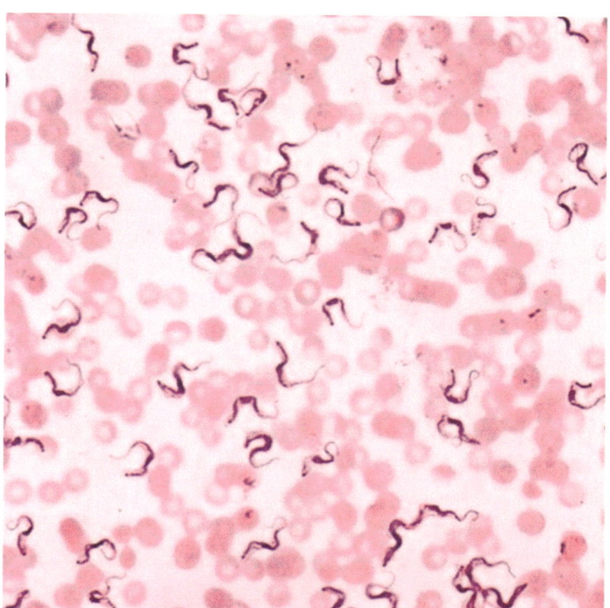

**Figure 2.**
*Flagellated tripoamastigote causing the circulating phase of the disease.*

It can be classified as asymptomatic, early symptoms (<less than 30 days old), or late symptoms (> 30 days old) [8].

The specific symptoms, which occur in the chronic stage, will depend directly on the organ that is affected and the damage that has occurred during the entire period of the disease. There is an asymptomatic chronic phase. This is characterized by the absence of symptoms and the presence of parasitemia and/or positive serology. This form can persist but only 30% of the patient the rest may progress to symptomatic form over a period of 10–30 years.

The symptomatic phase consists of the presence of chronic heart disease (cardiomegaly) represents the main cause of mortality and/or gastrointestinal disease (megaesophagus, megacolon, megaileum, megastomach, megabladder, megaduodenum, and megajejunum) with fluctuating parasitemia levels.

## 6. Chagasic megaesophagus

The most common gastrointestinal affectation due to Chagas disease is the megaesophagus, it affects any age, sex, and stage of the disease. The initial symptoms can be quite nonspecific, such as hypersalivation, nocturnal cough, a sensation of coughing after eating, and weight loss that further complicates the diagnosis [13], is characterized by the inability of the esophagus lower esophageal sphincter (LES) to relax in response to swallowing and absence of peristalsis in the esophageal body and; both motor abnormalities determine esophageal dilation with food stasis that will produce most of the symptoms and complications of the disease [13].

In the acute phase of the disease, parasites cause invasion of muscle tissue of the heart and digestive system, causing ganglionitis and lymphocytic infiltration, which leads to neuronal degeneration in these organs. It has been observed a massive loss of myenteric neurons, while the loss of submucosal neurons is moderate [14]. The asymptomatic or indeterminate chronic phase is clinically silent and with very low parasitemia, the duration varies between 5, 10, and up to 20 years; during this stage, the diagnostic methods of choice are serological tests. After this phase, the chronic symptomatic period occurs in which approximately 27% of patients present cardiac lesions, 6% damage to the digestive system (mainly in the esophagus and colon), and 3% to the peripheral nervous system [13].

The myenteric and submucosal plexus make up the enteric nervous system in humans, where the ganglionic nerve networks are located. The myenteric or Auerbach's plexus is located between the muscular layer and the longitudinal layer (**Figure 3**) and extends from the upper part of the esophagus to the internal anal sphincter. Additionally, the human submucosa contains two ganglion plexuses, the inner one is called Meissner's plexus and is localized in the submucosal plexus, while the Schabadasch's plexus is outer [15].

The progressive and irreversible deterioration in the enteric nervous system caused by the *T. cruzi* parasite is responsible for most of the gastrointestinal symptoms. Although any organ of the digestive system can be affected by Chagas disease, the esophagus and the colon are the ones that are most frequently damaged. The symptoms associated with Chagasic megaesophagus generally do not put the patient's pathway at risk, however, they considerably reduce their quality of life, since they generate eating disorders secondary to dysphagia, odynophagia, or esophageal insufficiency [16].

Hypocontractibility, motor dyskinesia, and incomplete or absent relaxation of the lower esophageal sphincter are results of this destruction of the myenteric plexuses,

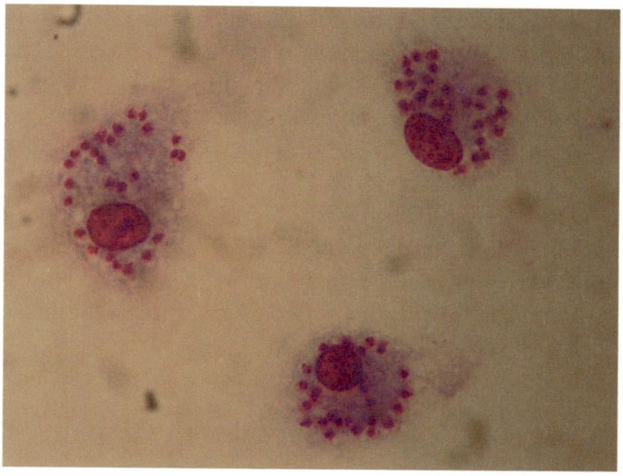

**Figure 3.**
*Amastigote without flagellum responsible for cell invasion.*

which lead to the classic presentation of achalasia. In esophageal symptoms and altered motility, an increase in the diameter of the esophagus is observed in 7–10% of infected subjects (Nisimura et al., 2020). Despite the findings that have been made in relation to the loss of esophageal motility secondary to damage to nerve structures, it has been proposed that the condition in other cell groups is necessary to explain more broadly the damage caused by the parasite. Therefore, it has been proposed that the damage caused to the muscle and nerve layers is also associated with immunomodulatory mechanisms and the local inflammatory response [14].

The biomechanics of swallowing is directly related to the contraction of the suprahyoid muscles. This contraction promotes the elevation and stabilization of the laryngeal complex during swallowing. Analysis of the suprahyoid musculature by electromyography has generally included the end of the oral phase, the pharyngeal

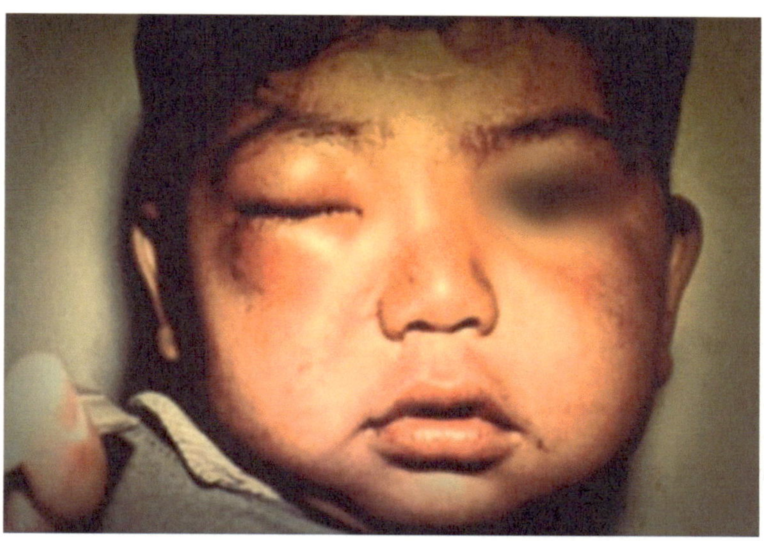

**Figure 4.**
*Unilateral eyelid edema, Romaña-Mazza sign.*

phase, and the beginning of the esophageal phase. In the oral and pharyngeal phases of swallowing in patients with Chagas disease, there is an increase in oral residues, a longer pharyngeal clearance and upper esophageal transit, and a longer opening of the upper esophageal sphincter. It has been observed that the contractile activity in the electromyography of patients with Chagas disease is lower than that of those who present motor esophageal disorders without this disease. This may be explained by decreased muscle recruitment of the suprahyoid muscles in patients with Chagasic megaesophagus and symptoms of dysphagia [16].

The diagnosis of Chagas megaesophagus is based mainly on the clinical history, symptoms, barium esophagram (**Figure 4**), manometry, and endoscopy [17], which could be classified as follows.

**Rezende's classification of Chagasic esophagopathy**

| Stage | Description |
|---|---|
| Stage 0 | indeterminate phase |
| Stage 1 | normal diameter with delayed emptying |
| Stage 2 | Moderate esophageal dilation and hypertonia of the lower esophageal sphincter |
| Stage 3 | Large increase in caliber with little contractile activity |
| Stage 4 | Megaesophagus |

An objective way to assess the severity of symptoms, as well as the effectiveness of treatment, is the Eckardt score, which ranges from 0 to 12 points, which classifies the stages of the disease. The score assigns from 0 to 3 for weight loss, dysphagia, chest pain, and regurgitation, the final value consisting of the sum of these elements—stage 0 (0–1 points), stage I (2–3 points), stage II (4–6 points), and stage III (> 6 points) [18].

**Eckardt Clinical Scoring System for Achalasia**

| Score | Weightloss | Dysphagia | Retrosternal chest pain | Regurgitation |
|---|---|---|---|---|
| 0 | No | No | No | No |
| 1 | < 5 kg | Often | Often | Often |
| 2 | 5-10 kg | Everyday | Everyday | Everyday |
| 3 | >10 kg | Each meal | Each meal | Each meal |

The goal of treatment is to restore the ability to feed orally and alleviate all these symptoms, which can be achieved by various modalities, such as endoscopic dilation, peri-oral endoscopic myotomy, and Heller Pinotti laparoscopic cardiomyotomy, which is currently considered the standard treatment for non-advanced megaesophagus patients. These modalities eliminate resistance to the outflow of food, improving esophageal emptying [18].

Recurrence of dysphagia after cardiomyotomy is associated with gastroesophageal reflux with esophagitis, incomplete myotomy, fibrosis at the site of the gastroesophageal junction, an inappropriate indication of technique for patients with advanced megaesophagus, and intrathoracic migration of the gastric fundus. The reoperation is usually not very successful in relation to the first procedure and many patients require esophagectomy treatment, which is the option of choice when symptoms reappear or the stage is advanced but adds greater morbidity and mortality associated with thoracic esophageal dissection. An alternative to esophagectomy is esophageal mucosectomy, with less morbidity due to preservation of the esophageal muscle tunica and an intraluminal dissection of the esophageal mucosa with subsequent transposition of the gastric tube without violation of the mediastinum [18].

The appropriate choice of surgical treatment for recurrent achalasia depends on the pathophysiology of the recurrence. Therefore, for patients with incomplete myotomy or fibrosis at the esophagogastric junction, a new myotomy with partial fundoplication is still indicated, as long as the esophageal wall has not been damaged during dissection. For patients with significant reflux or dolichomegaesophagus, the indication is esophagectomy with transposition of a stomach or colonic tube [18].

## 7. Chagasic megacolon

As previously described, this disease occurs in two phases, an acute one characterized by cell destruction, extensive inflammatory foci, and a large number of circulating parasites, and a chronic phase that can cause potentially fatal cardiac and digestive disorders [19]. It has been described that up to 40% of people who suffer from it will develop one of these complications or a combination of both [20]. Megacolon is defined as irreversible dilation of the colonic segment, predominantly in the chronic phase of Chagas disease, where the dilated segment presents histopathological changes characterized by a significant loss of neurons of the myenteric or Auerbach and submucosal or Meissner plexus and although not the mechanisms of this destruction are well elucidated, it has been proposed that it could be due to the release of toxins during the fragmentation of the parasite, direct cellular damage, or inflammatory damage [20, 21].

Recently it has been described that the progress to the chronic phase is determined mainly by an inflammatory state, to which the virulence of the parasite and its tropism for the tissues contribute. During Chagasic cardiomyopathy, there is an extensive production of pro-inflammatory cytokines, such as interferon γ (INF γ), Tumor Necrosis Factor α (TNF α), as well as other mechanisms that cause tissue damage, such as the cytotoxic activity of CD8 T lymphocytes [10]. Similarly, in Chagasic megacolon, the myenteric plexus is severely affected by an inflammatory process that leads to neuronal degeneration, ganglionitis, peri-ganglionitis, neuritis, and peri-neuritis. The inflammatory infiltrate has been characterized by the presence of eosinophils, mast cells, CD68 + macrophages, Natural Killer CD57 + cells, and TIA-1 + cytotoxic lymphocytes that maintain the inflammatory process and neuronal destruction [21]. It has also been described that the neuronal destruction process derives from an autoimmune response mediated mainly by TNF α and INF γ. Both cytokines are involved in the control of the parasite during acute infection, however, an imbalance in the response of these cytokines can lead to progression to chronicity and eventually to the cardiac and intestinal complications characteristic of the chronic phase of the disease [21]. The role of the megacolon in the context of intestinal neoplasms is controversial. It is suggested that derived from the dilation of the organ and the presence of food stasis, there is prolonged contact between the intestinal mucosa and potentially carcinogenic agents. In this context, the role of Galectin 3, a protein whose increased expression is related to tumor progression and which is used by *T. cruzi* to enter cells, has been studied, which suggests that there could be a relationship between this protein and neoplastic progression [22]. However, other studies have sought to demonstrate that patients with chronic-phase Chagas disease have a lower risk of colon tumors at least in the megacolon region, probably derived from denervation in this area, since it has been proposed that neuronal invasion could promote tumor invasion [23].

According to current estimates, up to 10,000 deaths associated with this disease could occur annually [24], since between 15 and 20% of all cases will present digestive complications, including megaesophagus and megacolon [25]. The prevalence of megacolon in patients with Chagas disease may be higher in those who presented symptoms during the acute phase than in those in whom there were no manifestations in this phase [26].

Chagasic megacolon presents clinically with chronic constipation due to pathological dilation of the organ wall, mainly in the sigmoid portion of the colon, a site where *T. cruzi* is commonly found [27]. This is considered to be the most frequent symptom in patients with Chagasic megacolon, however, it has been reported that there are patients with normal evacuations, as well as patients with Chagas disease who present constipation not associated with megacolon.

Although this sequel is well known in the context of Chagas disease, few studies have described the clinical manifestations of its presentation, having little information on digestive visceromegaly caused by *T. cruzi*. In some case reports, constipation is reported as well as other associated signs and symptoms, such as bloating [28]. Likewise, it has been described those subjects with megacolon present a decrease in basal motility and wave frequency in manometry, absence of an inhibitory rectus-anal reflex, and it is noteworthy that in patients with diverticular disease and Chagasic megacolon, the diverticula appear in non-dilated portions of the colon [29].

The approach to patients with megacolon associated with Chagas disease is complex because most infected patients do not present symptoms in the acute phase; so, it is very likely that they will seek care when the typical manifestations of megacolon appear (constipation, abdominal pain, diarrhea, changes in defecatory habits, or bloody stools); in this situation, if the patient is not known to have trypanosomiasis and lives in an endemic area, it will be essential to make a proper diagnosis of this disease [30, 31]. When questioning these patients, other associated symptoms and signs should be identified, since heart disease coexists in up to 30% of cases. Likewise, it is necessary to question the patient about other digestive symptoms, since some of these are not associated with Chagas disease [30]. In the study of patients in the chronic phase, the diagnostic methods are indirect, that is, laboratory techniques that identify antigens of *T. cruzi* (direct hemagglutination) or antibodies against the parasite (Enzyme Immuno Assay, Indirect Immunofluorescence, Western Blot) [31].

The diagnosis of megacolon depends on clinical, radiological, endoscopic, and surgical findings. One of the most widely used radiological studies is the Barium enema or colon enema (**Figure 5**), with which the diagnosis can be confirmed if the rectosigmoid diameter at the pelvic border is greater than 6.5 cm or the diameter of the middle sigmoid is 10 cm or more. Computed tomography colonography can also be used as it allows measurement of the diameters and length of the colon from different views [32]. Colonoscopy is not the ideal study for the identification of megacolon, since it depends on the interpretation of the person who performs it, in this sense, the diagnosis can be made through the result of incomplete colonoscopy [32].

The management of megacolon will depend on the degree of constipation of the patient, his/her nutritional status, and his/her comorbidities. Treatment options are clinical or symptomatic and surgical. There is no consensus on the surgical management of choice, however, the most widely used procedure is the Duhamel-Haddad

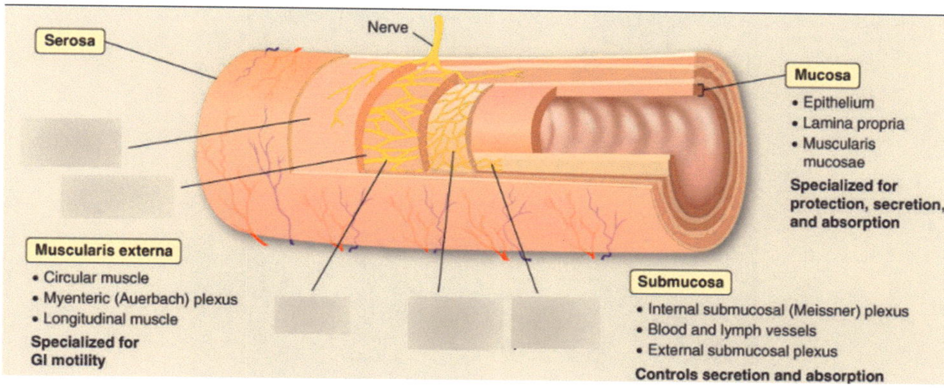


**Figure 5.**
*Nervous plexuses of the digestive system.*

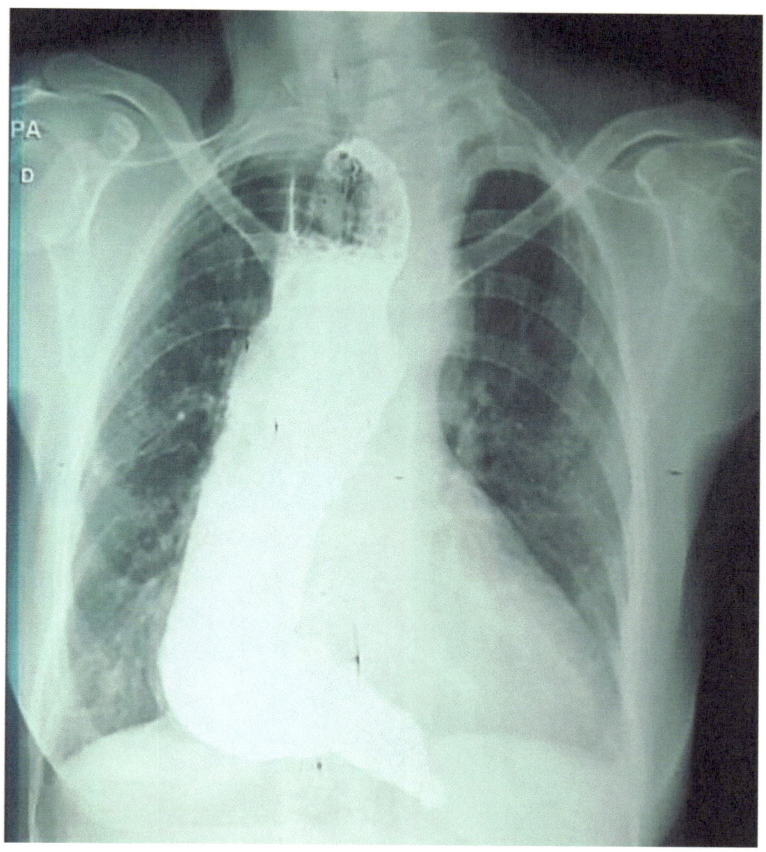


**Figure 6.**
*Megaesophagus seen with barium esophagram.*

procedure (rectosigmoidectomy with retrocecal interposition) or rectosigmoidectomy with low end-to-side colorectal anastomosis (see **Figures 6–8**) [30].

It has been reported that complications derived from chronic constipation such as rectal prolapse or acute volvulus may occur [32, 33] (imagen 8). Of these, the most

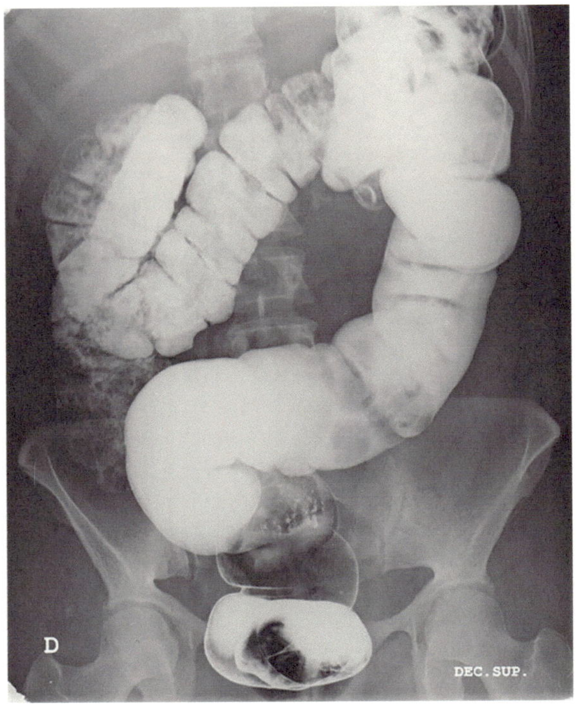


**Figure 7.**
*Barium enema showing megacolon.*

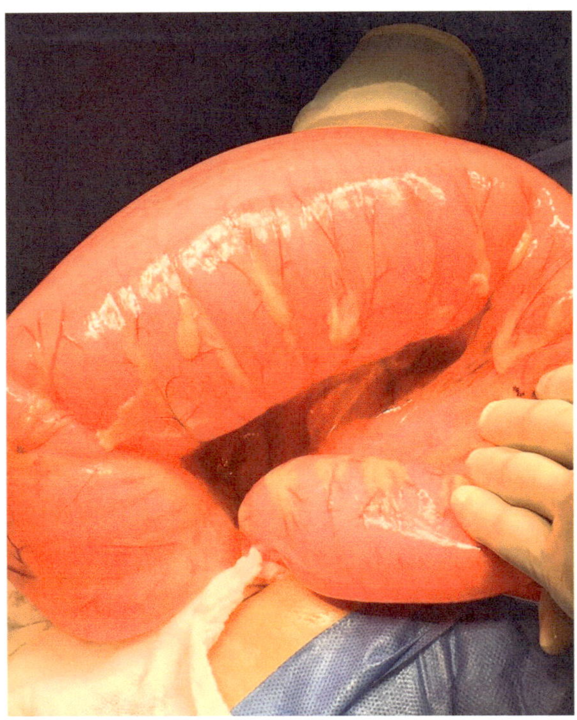

**Figure 8.**
*Intraoperative image of sigmoid volvulation in chagasic megacolon.*

serious complication is volvulus, which occurs when a redundant loop of the colon rotates around the mesentery, which, in turn, causes a closed-loop intestinal obstruction that generates ischemia due to hypoperfusion of the affected segment, where there is an accumulation of gas associated with fermentation of intestinal contents. When this happens, the tension of the wall increases, which worsens the ischemia and promotes perforation of the intestine, which could lead to the death of the patient [34].

The treatment of volvulus is based on the control of symptoms and resuscitation of the patient and then decompression and derotation of the intestine by endoscopy if there is no evidence of peritonitis or perforation, since, if it occurs, the treatment is invariably urgent surgical [34].

## 8. Conclusion

American trypanosomiasis is one of the most serious parasitic diseases in the world, it has economic implications in public health systems that condition costs for complications in the different body systems, as well as loss of working years when diagnosed mainly in asymptomatic chronic stages. Damage to the digestive system due to the destruction of neuronal plexuses is responsible for most of the symptoms in chronic stages, which condition disability and put the patient's life at risk, so early diagnosis in acute stages is the main tool to stop this disease.

## Author details

Víctor Hugo García Orozco*, Juan Enrique Villalvazo Navarro, Carlos Solar Aguirre, Carlos Manuel Ibarra Ocampo, César Iván Díaz Sandoval, Carlos Alejandro Ortíz Gallegos, Diego Javier Oregel Camacho and Araceli Noriega Bucio
Hospital Civil de Tepic "Dr. Antonio González Guevara", Tepic, Nayarit, México

*Address all correspondence to: victor-garcia.cirugia@hotmail.com

## References

[1] García-Orozco VH, García-Sánchez D, López-Flores JF, Sánchez-Mata R. Pediatric sigmoid volvulus due to Chagas disease. Cir y Cir (English Ed.). 2019;**87**(5):568-571

[2] Marcelo D, Rocha MC, María D, Sarubbi A. Presentacion De Un Caso Clinico y Revision Bibliografica. Minerva: 29-35

[3] Frisancho VO. Dolicomegacolon andino y vólvulos intestinales de altura: [revisión]. Rev Gastroenterol del Perú. 2008;**28**(3):248-257

[4] Saravia Burgos J, Acosta CA. Megacolon y vólvulo de sigmoides: incidencia y fisiopatología. Revista de Gastroenterología del Perú. 2015;**35**(1):38-44

[5] Chao C, Leone JL, Vigliano CA. Chagas disease: Historic perspective. Biochimical Biophysics Acta - Molecular Basis Dis. 2020;**1866**(5)

[6] Steverding D. The history of Chagas disease. Parasites and Vectors. 2014;**7**(1):1-8

[7] Hubbert S. Simulation models. Essent Math Mark Risk Management. 2012;**13**(4):291-307

[8] Álvarez-HernándezD,Franyuti-KellyG, Díaz-López-Silva R, González-Chávez A, GonzálezHermosillo-Cornejo D, Vázquez-López R. Chagas disease: Current perspectives on a forgotten disease. Rev Med Hosp Gen Méx. 2018;**81**(3):154-164. DOI: 10.1016/j.hgmx.2016.09.010

[9] Zingales B, Miles MA, Campbell DA, Tibayrenc M, Macedo AM, Teixeira MMG, et al. The revised *Trypanosoma cruzi* subspecific nomenclature: Rationale, epidemiological relevance and research applications. Infection, Genetics and Evolution. 2012;**12**(2):240-253. DOI: 10.1016/j.meegid.2011.12.009

[10] Pérez-Molina JA, Molina I. Chagas disease. Lancet. 2018;**391**(10115):82-94

[11] Murcia L, Carrilero B, Munoz-Davila MJ, Thomas MC, López MC, Segovia M. Risk factors and primary prevention of congenital chagas disease in a nonendemic country. Clinical Infectious Diseases. 2013;**56**(4):496-502

[12] Flávia Nardy A, Freire-De-Lima CG, Morrot A. Immune evasion strategies of *Trypanosoma cruzi*. Journal of Immunology Research. 2015;**2015**

[13] Carod-Artal FJ. Infectious diseases causing autonomic dysfunction. Clinical Autonomic Research. 2018;**28**(1):67-81

[14] Nisimura LM, Coelho LL, de Melo TG, de Vieira PC, Victorino PH, Garzoni LR, et al. *Trypanosoma cruzi* promotes transcriptomic remodeling of the JAK/STAT signaling and cell cycle pathways in myoblasts. Frontiers in Cellular and Infection Microbiology. 2020;**10**(June):1-15

[15] Martins P, Ferreira CS, Cunha-Melo JR. Esophageal transit time in patients with chagasic megaesophagus. Medicine (Baltimore). 2018;**97**(10):e0084

[16] El Gharib AZG, Berretin-Felix G, Dantas RO, Rossoni DF, de Ornelas Toledo MJ. Suprahyoid muscle activity in patients with chagasic megaesophagus. Scientific Reports. 2019;**9**(1):1-7

[17] De Barros F, De Almeida Soares JC, De Barros FP, Conde Sangenis LH, Da Silva GMS, Monteiro Fonseca AB, et al. Agreement between upper endoscopy and esophagography in the diagnosis of megaesophagus in Chagas disease. Revista da Sociedade Brasileira de Medicina Tropical. 2019;**52**:1-5

[18] Costa LCDS, Braga JGR, Tercioti Junior V, de Neto JSC, Ferrer JAP, Lopes LR, et al. Surgical treatment of relapsed megaesophagus. Revista do Colégio Brasileiro de Cirurgiões. 2020;**47**(1):1-7

[19] Do Carmo Neto JR, Braga YLL, Da Costa AWF, Lucio FH, Do Nascimento TC, Dos Reis MA, et al. Biomarkers and their possible functions in the intestinal microenvironment of chagasic megacolon: An overview of the (neuro)inflammatory process. Journal of Immunology Research. 2021;**2021**

[20] Rassi A, Rassi A, Marin-Neto JA. Chagas disease. Lancet. 2010;**375**(9723): 1388-1402. DOI: 10.1016/S0140-6736 (10)60061-X

[21] Jabari S, De Oliveira EC, Brehmer A, Da Silveira ABM. Chagasic megacolon: Enteric neurons and related structures. Histochemistry and Cell Biology. 2014;**142**(3):235-244

[22] Garvil MP, de Furtado TCS, de Lima NB, Marteleto MVM, de Faria JB, Rodrigues DBR, et al. Although with intact mucosa at colonoscopy, chagasic megacolons have an overexpression of Gal-3. Einstein (Sao Paulo). 2020;**18**:eAO5105

[23] Kannen V, de Oliveira EC, Motta BZ, Chaguri AJ, Brunaldi MO, Garcia SB. Trypanosomiasis-induced megacolon illustrates how myenteric neurons modulate the risk for colon cancer in rats and humans. PLoS Neglected Tropical Diseases. 2015;**9**(4):1-12

[24] Stanaway JD, Roth G. The burden of Chagas disease estimates and challenges. Global Heart. 2015;**10**(3):139-144. DOI: 10.1016/j.gheart.2015.06.001

[25] Teixeira ARL, Nitz N, Guimaro MC, Gomes C, Santos-Buch CA. Chagas disease. Postgraduate Medical Journal. 2006;**82**(974):788-798

[26] Castro C, Bernal Hernandez E, Rezende J, Prata A. Estudo radiológico do megacólon em área endêmica de doença de Chagas Radiological study on megacolon cases in an endemic area for Chagas disease. Revista da Sociedade Brasileira de Medicina Tropical. 2010;**43**(5):562-566

[27] Bafutto M, Luquetti AO, Gabriel Neto S, Penhavel FAS, Oliveira EC. Constipation is related to small bowel disturbance rather than colonic enlargement in acquired chagasic megacolon. Gastroenterology Research. 2017;**10**(4):213-217

[28] Adad SJ, Etchebehere RM, de Araujo JR, Madureira AB, Lima VGF, da Silva AA, et al. Association of chagasic megacolon and cancer of the colon: Case report and review of the literature. Revista da Sociedade Brasileira de Medicina Tropical. 2002;**35**(1):63-68

[29] Matsuda NM, Miller SM, Evora PRB. The chronic gastrointestinal manifestations of chagas disease. Clinics. 2009;**64**(12):1219-1224

[30] Pinazo MJ, Cañas EG, Elizalde JI, García M, Gascón J, Gimeno F, et al. Diagnosis, management and treatment of chronic chagas' gastrointestinal disease in areas where *Trypanosoma cruzi* infection is not endemic. Gastroenterología y Hepatología. 2010;**33**(3):191-200

[31] Secretaría de Salud Dirección General de Epidemiología. Manual de

Procedimientos Estandarizados para la Vigilancia Epidemiológica de las Enfermedades Transmitidas por Vector (ETV). Manual ETV´s 2020 - Dirección General de Epidemiología. 2021. p. 1375. Available from: https://epidemiologia.salud.gob.mx

[32] Cuda T, Gunnarsson R, de Costa A. Symptoms and diagnostic criteria of acquired megacolon—A systematic literature review. BMC Gastroenterology. 2018;**18**(1):1-9

[33] Lara-Romero C, Ferreiro-Argüelles B, Romero-Pérez E. Complicaciones colónicas agudas en paciente con enfermedad de Chagas. Rev. esp. enferm. Dig. 2016;**12**(108):841-842

[34] Melling J, Makin CA. Sigmoid volvulus, acquired megacolon and pseudo-obstruction. Surgery. 2011;**29**(8):387-390. DOI: 10.1016/j.mpsur.2011.05.019

Chapter 6

# How Do Mouse Strains and Inoculation Routes Influence the Course of Experimental *Trypanosoma cruzi* Infection?

*Flávia de Oliveira Cardoso, Carolina Salles Domingues, Tânia Zaverucha do Valle and Kátia da Silva Calabrese*

## Abstract

Chagas' disease outcomes depend on several factors including parasite and host genetics, immune response, and route of infection. In this study, we investigate the influence of inoculation route and host genetic background on the establishment and development of Chagas disease in mice, using an isolate of *Trypanosoma cruzi* SC2005 strain (TcII), which was obtained from an oral Chagas' disease outbreak in Santa Catarina, Brazil. Comparative analysis of the immunopathological, histopathological, and hematological profiles of mice was performed demonstrating the influence of the route of infection in disease severity. In outbred mice, intraperitoneal (IP) infection led to higher infection and mortality rates and more severe parasitaemia, when compared with intragastric (IG) infection. Nevertheless, tissue colonization was similar, showing severe damage in the heart, with intense lymphocytic inflammatory infiltrates, regardless of the route of infection. On the other hand, in mice IG-infected, the host genetic background influences the start timing of immune response against *Trypanosoma cruzi*. The susceptible BALB/c inbred mouse strain presented an earlier development of a cytotoxic cellular profile, when compared with A mice. We hypothesize that the cytotoxic response mounted before the parasitaemia increase allowed for a milder manifestation of Chagas' disease in intragastrically infected mice.

**Keywords:** Chagas disease, immunopathology, host genetics, inoculation route, mice

## 1. Introduction

Chagas' disease is a public health problem that affects about 6 to 7 million people worldwide, mainly who reside in the endemic areas of 21 countries of Latin America [1]. Despite the progress made to control the infection, the disease has been expanding to North America, Europe, Australia, and Japan by migration of million people from endemic countries [2–4]. The etiological agent of disease is the protozoan *Trypanosoma cruzi*, which shows a wide genetic variation, being classified in seven Discrete Typing Units (DTUs), TcI–TcVI, and Tcbat [5–7]. These different DTUs are responsible for different disease outcomes, demonstrating the influence of parasite genetics on disease development [6]. Chagas' disease is classically transmitted by its insect vector, the triatomine bugs [8], but can also be acquired by blood transfusion [9, 10], congenitally [11, 12], by organ transplantation [13, 14], laboratory accidents [15], sexually [16], and by ingestion of contaminated food/juice [17]. After successful actions to interrupt vector transmission, oral contamination has been considered the main route of transmission in several countries [17–19]. Brazil is the country with the highest incidence of oral acute Chagas' disease outbreaks, mainly in the Amazon Basin ([19] reviewed by [20]). Oral acute Chagas' disease displays a higher number of signs and symptoms and higher lethality than those acquired through the vectorial route [17, 21].

In addition to parasite genetics and route of infection, disease outcome is also influenced by other factors such as evolutive forms of the parasite, parasite load, mixed infections [22–25], and host factors including immune response, concomitant infections, nutrition deficiencies, and host genetics [26]. Although several studies have tried to identify the genetic basis of Chagas disease, our knowledge on the subject is still vague. Many works have studied genetic polymorphisms located in genes associated with immune response [27] or over the whole genome [28, 29], but the influence of these polymorphisms on the pathology of the disease still needs to be further validated.

Considering the complexity of these factors and their influence in Chagas' disease immunopathogenesis, anti-*Trypanosoma cruzi* immune response and chemotherapy, there is a need to improve our understanding about these relationships. On this way, this study investigates the influence of the inoculation route and the host genetic background on the establishment and development of Chagas' disease in inbred and outbred mice, using an isolate of *T. cruzi* SC2005 strain (TcII) obtained from a human case from an oral Chagas' disease outbreak in the south region of Brazil [30]. The aim was to conduct a comparative analysis of the immunopathological, histopathological and hematological profiles, using parameters such as parasite load, survival rates, cytokines production, histopathology, and cell populations in the inflammatory sites.

## 2. Materials and methods

### 2.1 Ethics statement

All experiments were conducted following the guidelines for experimental procedures of the National Council for the Control of Animal Experimentation (CONCEA) after approval by the Ethics Committee for Animal Research of the Fundação Oswaldo Cruz (CEUA-FIOCRUZ) under licenses number LW16/11 (Swiss Webster mice) and LW 42/14 (A and BALB/c mice).

### 2.2 Animals

BALB/c, A and Swiss Webster female mice, 4–6 weeks old, were provided by Instituto de Ciência e Tecnologia em Biomodelos (ICTB - FIOCRUZ) and housed under pathogen-free conditions, controlled temperature, and food and water *ad libitum*.

### 2.3 Parasites

*Trypanosoma cruzi* SC2005 (DTU Tc II), isolated from a case of oral acute Chagas' disease during an outbreak in Santa Catarina, Brazil [30, 31], was used in this study.

In experiments with outbred Swiss mice, epimastigote forms of *T. cruzi* SC2005 isolate were maintained in LIT medium for 30 days. Metacyclic trypomastigotes forms were quantified in a Neubauer chamber and used to infect VERO cells. The infected culture was maintained in RPMI medium, supplemented with 10% fetal bovine serum. Trypomastigotes derived from cell culture (TCC) were obtained 10 days after, by recovering parasites from the culture supernatant, and quantified in a Neubauer chamber prior to infecting mouse groups.

In experiments with inbred mice (A and BALB/c), epimastigote forms were maintained at 28°C for 21 days in LIT (Liver Infusion, Triptose) (AGM) culture medium to obtained metacyclic forms that were quantified in a Neubauer hemocytometer prior to infection.

### 2.4 Experimental design

In order to investigate the influence of the route of infection on the course of *T. cruzi* SC2005 infection, Swiss mice were organized into three groups: group 1 (n = 30) mice intraperitoneally (IP) infected by $10^7$ TCC forms of *T. cruzi* SC2005 strain/0.2 mL of RPMI medium; group 2 (n = 55) mice intragastrically infected by $10^7$ TCC forms of *T. cruzi* SC2005 strain/0.1 mL of RPMI medium using a gavage needle (subjected to 4 h of fasting prior to infection), and group 3 (n = 15) normal uninfected animals (control group). Mice from each group (n = 3) were euthanized at 11 and 18 (IP-infected mice) and 26 and 33 (IG-infected mice) days after infection, and the esophagus, stomach, intestines, heart, thymus, liver, spleen, pancreas, kidney, adrenal gland, bladder, uterus, mesenteric lymph nodes, and brain were removed.

In experiments to investigate the host genetics influence on the course of *T. cruzi* SC2005 infection, A and BALB/c mice were intragastrically infected by $10^7$ metacyclic trypomastigote forms of *T. cruzi* SC2005 strain/0.3 mL of LIT medium using a gavage needle. Prior to intragastric injection, the animals were submitted to 4 h of fasting. The animals were divided into four experimental groups: Group 1 (n = 70): A-infected mice; Group 2 (n = 70) BALB/c-infected, and Group 3 (n = 50) and Group 4 (n = 50)—each one composed by uninfected A and BALB/c mice (control groups), respectively. Mice from each group (n = 6) were euthanized at 7-, 14-, 21-, and 40-day post-infection (dpi), and the blood, esophagus, stomach, gut, heart, and liver were removed.

### 2.5 Parasitemia, mortality and leukometry

Ten mice of each infected group were monitored daily from 5 to 50 dpi. Parasitaemia was determined as described by Pizzi and Prager [32]. Briefly, 5 μL of blood's tail vein was collected and placed under a cover slip (22 x 22 mm) and the number of parasites/mL of blood was estimated by counting 50 microscopic fields in a 400X magnification. Mice that did not develop parasitaemia were considered non-infected and excluded from the experiment.

Mortality rate was estimated to obtain the survivors percentage. Mean time of death was calculated following Liddell [33].

At the same time of parasitaemia evaluation, another 10 μL of blood's tail vein was collected and diluted in Turk's solution (1/20) [34] for white cells counting using a Neubauer chamber. Differential cell count was made in smears, after MayGrünwald–Giemsa staining, by counting 100 leukocytes/slide.

## 2.6 Spleen index

Spleen index was calculated to investigate reticuloendothelial stimulation. This index was calculated after evaluation of the relative spleen weight (spleen weight/mouse weight) [35].

## 2.7 Parasite load

Fragments of heart recovered from infected mice were immediately frozen after euthanasia and stored at −70°C. Fragments were digested in 500 μL of lysis buffer (50 mM Tris, 10 mM NaCL, 5 mM EDTA, 0.5% SDS) containing proteinase K (20 mg/ml). DNA was extracted following a standard phenol/chloroform protocol [36]. DNA concentrations and purity were determined by reading A260 and A280 on a NanoDrop 2000c spectrophotometer (Thermo Fisher Scientific, Wilmington, DE, USA).

Parasite DNA was detected by SYBR Green qPCR assay using StepOnePlus Real-Time PCR System (Applied Biosystems). Primers targeting *T. cruzi* genomic DNA sequence (166 bp) Cruzi 1 (5'-ASTCGGCTGATCGTTTTCGA-3′) and Cruzi 2 (5'-AATTCCTCCAAGCAGCGGATA-3′) and Actb-actin, beta (b-actin) mouse gene (138 bp) (Forward 5'-AGAGGGAAATCGTGCGTGAC-3′; reverse 5'CAATAGTGATGACCTGGCCGT3') were used following previous reports [37, 38]. To monitor DNA integrity, variation in DNA yield, or the presence of potential inhibitors of PCR, Actb reference gene was used as a positive control. The reaction mixtures contained Power SYBR Green PCR Master Mix 2X (Applied Biosystems), 25 ng of DNA template, and 100 nM of b-actin or 300 nM of Cruzi1/Cruzi2 primers in a final volume of 20 μL. PCR conditions were as follows: hold at 95°C for 10 min, 95°C for 15 s, and 58°C for 1 min (40x). Standard curves from axenic epimastigotes *T. cruzi* DNA (100 ng–1 pg) were generated. A melt curve analysis was performed on all reactions. The results were analyzed with the StepOne software v2.2.2 (Applied Biosystems).

## 2.8 Histopathology

Following euthanasia, all removed organs were fixed in 4% paraformaldehyde in phosphate-buffered saline (PBS), pH 7.45, at 4°C, for 72 h, cleaved and routinely processed paraffin embedded. Tissue sections (5 μm) were stained with Hematoxylin–Eosin (HE) (Sigma-Aldrich, Saint Louis, USA), Lennert's Giemsa, or Picro-Sirius red (Direct Red 80, Aldrich Milwaukee, WI 53233, USA) techniques. The presence of inflammatory infiltrates was classified as (−) without infiltrates, (+) very mild lesion areas, (++) mild lesion areas, (+++) moderate areas of infiltrates, (+++) severe areas of infiltrates, (++++) very severe areas of infiltrates, following described by Barreto-de-Albuquerque et al. [39], and arbitrary values from 0 to 5 were attributed to it. Tissues were analyzed and photographed under light microscopy (Zeiss, Axioplan 2, with Axiovision LE64 photomicrograph equipment).

### 2.9 Hemogram

The blood was collected by cardiac puncture, placed in EDTA tubes, and sent to the Laborlife clinical laboratory (RJ, Brazil). Complete blood count (CBC) was analyzed in an automatic cell counter (Beckman Coulter, Brea, CA). The blood parameters evaluated were red blood cell (RBC), hemoglobin (Hgb), hematocrit (Hct), mean corpuscular volume (MCV), mean corpuscular hemoglobin (MCH), mean corpuscular hemoglobin concentration (MCHC), white blood cell (WBC), and platelet (PLT).

### 2.10 Cytokine analysis

Detection of TNF-$\alpha$, IFN-$\gamma$, IL-10, IL-6, IL-17A, IL-4, and IL-2 was performed through BD Cytometric Bead Array (CBA) Mouse Th1/Th2/Th17 Cytokine Kit (cat. 560,485; BD Biosciences, San Jose, CA) following manufacturer's instructions. Samples were acquired in the BD Q13 FACSCallibur flow cytometer (BD Biosciences) and data were analyzed with FCAP Array software (BD Biosciences).

### 2.11 Obtaining of mononuclear cells to flow cytometry

In the determined euthanasia points, the blood of each animal was collected by cardiac puncture using citrated saline (0.87% NaCl, 3.8% $Na_3C_6H_5O_7$) and diluted in the same volume of complete RPMI medium—RPMI 1640 medium (Sigma-Aldrich, St. Louis, MO), supplemented with 10% fetal bovine serum (FBS) (CultiLab, Campinas, Brazil); 200 mM L-glutamine; 100 U/mL penicillin; and 10 mg/mL streptomycin (Sigma-Aldrich, St. Louis, MO). Cells were then added to a Ficoll–Hypaque (Histopaque 1077; Sigma-Aldrich) sedimentation gradient. After centrifugation at 1030 x g for 20 min at 21 C, without brake, the mononuclear cell (MCs) ring was collected. A lobe of the liver, mesenteric lymph nodes, and spleen were macerated in 4 mL of complete RPMI medium until complete disruption using a glass tissue homogenizer (Corning E.U.A.), being kept on ice throughout the process. Cardiac cells were obtained after organ perfusion with PBS (pH 7.2), subsequently cut into small fragments, and subjected to four cycles of dissociation using 0.2% type II collagenase in RPMI medium without FBS at 37°C, stirring for 30 min. The supernatant obtained after each dissociation cycle was collected in a single tube and kept on ice. Cells from blood, liver, spleen, mesenteric lymph nodes, and heart were washed twice (with centrifugation at 720 x g, 4°C, 5 min) in PBS-BSA-(Bovine Serum Albumin) with 10% FBS and resuspended with 3 mL of ACK (Ammonium-Chloride-Potassium) Lysing Buffer, to lyse of red blood cells, incubated for 5 min at room temperature and washed again. After that, cells were incubated in PBS-BSA with 10% horse serum (HS) for 30 min, washed again, resuspended with complete RPMI medium, and adjusted to $1x10^6$cells/well.

### 2.12 Flow cytometry

Cells were incubated for 20 min in the dark at room temperature with the following monoclonal-antibody panel: anti-CD3-PC7 (Cat 553,064; BD Biosciences—maximum emission (max-em): 785 nm) diluted 1:40; anti-CD4-APC-H7 (Cat 560,181; BD Biosciences—max-em: 785 nm) diluted 1:80; anti-CD8-BB515 (Cat. 564,422; BD Biosciences—max-em: 515 nm) diluted 1:160, and anti-CD19-APC (Cat MCA 1439;

Serotec—max-em: 661 nm) diluted 1:20, in PBS-BSA-HS. Cells were washed with PBS to remove unbound antibodies, fixed in 1% paraformaldehyde for 30 min in the dark at 4°C, washed again, and stored at 4°C in the dark until acquisition in flow cytometry. At least 20,000 events from each sample were acquired through CytoFlex flow cytometer (Beckman Coulter). Single-stained controls were used to set compensation parameters, while unstained cells were used to set analysis regions. After acquisition, flow cytometric analysis to evaluate the frequencies of $CD8^{+}$T, $CD4^{+}$T, $CD4^{+}/CD8^{+}$ T, and $CD19^{+}$B cells was performed using CytoExpert Software (Beckman Coulter). A gate strategy was performed as follows: to exclude cell aggregates from analyses, cells were gated on Singlets region in FSC-A vs. FSC-H dot-plot; from Singlets gate an FSC-A vs. Side-Scatter-Area (SSCA), dot plot was created and the analyses region (mononuclear cells) was defined to encompass mononuclear cells and exclude dead cells from analyses; from Mono gate, $CD4^{+}$ and $CD8^{+}$ T lymphocytes were determined by CD3 vs. CD4 and CD3 vs. CD8 dot plots, respectively, and $CD19^{+}$B cells by CD3 vs. CD19 dot plot. $CD4^{+}/CD8^{+}$ double-positive T cells was determined by plotting CD8 vs. CD4 gated on $CD3^{+}$.

### 2.13 Statistical analysis

Data are expressed by mean ± standard error of the mean (SEM) and analyzed statistically by two- or one-way ANOVA and Sidak's multiple comparison post-test using the GraphPad Prism 6 software. Differences were considered significant when $p < 0.05$.

## 3. Results and discussion

### 3.1 Route of infection and host genetic background influence on the parasitaemia and mortality after *T. cruzi* SC2005 infection

Several studies have been showing that the course and severity of Chagas' disease depends on varied factors, among them are the route of infection and host genetic background [25].

The most frequent route of Chagas' transmission is currently by ingestion of contaminated food and beverages, especially in Brazil and some other endemic countries [19, 40–42]. Infection by oral route usually leads to a more severe acute disease than vector-borne infection. The amount of metacyclic trypomastigotes contained in a triatomine crushed in food or beverage may be more than 100 times higher than what is typically found on its feces [43]. Furthermore, the digestive mucosa represents an extensive gateway, containing different molecules that serve as attachment points to the parasite [44]. Therefore, orally infected patients tend to experience a more severe acute phase, with more rapid progression to long-term cardiac or gastrointestinal dysfunction and higher mortality [43]. In the experimental model, intraperitoneal inoculation is the most common route of infection, but it does not mimic any natural infection. It delivers elevated loads of trypomastigotes directly in the peritoneum, bypassing all natural barriers in the skin and mucosa. When mucosa and systemic *T. cruzi* infection were compared, distinct disease patterns can be observed. Several studies in mice showed that intraperitoneal infection induces higher parasitemia and mortality than intragastric (IG) or oral infection with the same inoculum [39, 45, 46]. Marsden [47] showed that systemic infections (intraperitoneal or intravenous) promote higher

DOI: http://dx.doi.org/10.5772/intechopen.104461

infection rates (67–100%) and mortality than mucosal (oral, intragastric, intrarectal, genitalia, or conjunctival infection) (17–67%) in mice infected by the Peruvian strain. In the present study, similar results were obtained when outbred Swiss mice were infected IG or IP with TCC forms of SC2005 *T. cruzi* strain. IP infection was able to infect 100% of animals, while just 36% of IG-infected mice developed parasitaemia. Moreover, IP-infected mice showed earlier (10th and 13th days) and higher parasitaemia peaks (2.9 and 4.3 X $10^6$ parasites/mL, respectively) than those observed in the IG-infected animals, which presented peaks on the 13th and 18th dpi with 0.9 and 1.7 X $10^6$ parasites/mL, respectively (**Figure 1A**). Furthermore, IP-infected animals died earlier (mean time of death of 16.13 ± 0.8 days), and its mortality rate was 80%. On the other hand, IG-infected mice died later (22.67 ± 2.0), and the mortality rate was around 30% (**Figure 1B**). Different infection routes submit parasites to different barriers in order to infect the host. Crossing of these barriers may explain the differences observed in course and intensity of the parasitaemia. Nevertheless, independent of the route of infection, parasites were able to make their way to the heart, which showed amastigote nests after infection by both routes (**Figure 1C** and **D**).

The success of *T. cruzi* infection and the level of parasitaemia after oral contamination are mainly determined by the magnitude of the mucosal immune response developed [48], which depends on the interaction between both parasite and host genetics [49, 50]. Studies of genetic susceptibility to Chagas' disease are scarce and its contribution to disease pathology is still unsolved. Inbred mice from different genetic backgrounds have been used to assess the influence of host genetics to several pathogens. Studies using inbred mouse strains infected by *T. cruzi* showed different profiles of response to infection and degrees of susceptibility in the hosts, with differences in mortality rate, cytokine production, inflammatory infiltrate, and parasite load [51–53]. C57BL/10 mice infected with *T. cruzi* SC2005 strain showed lower parasitaemia and mortality rate, while CBA-infected mice showed high parasitaemia and mortality rate [52]. Other studies using different inbred mouse strains (A/J, BALB/c, C3H/HePas, C57BL/6, and DBA mice) infected with *T. cruzi* Y also showed differences in mortality rate and parasitaemia. C57BL/6 mice were less susceptible to infection, while A/J was the most susceptible strain, showing the highest parasitemia and mortality rate [51]. In this work, we also observed significant differences in both parasite load and mortality rate between two mouse strains intragastrically infected with *T. cruzi* SC2005. The A mice were less susceptible to infection, showing lower parasitaemia (**Figure 2A**), parasite load in the heart (**Figure 2B**), and mortality rates (**Figure 2C**). Although these animals presented an earlier mortality (23 dpi), only 10% of the infected mice died. On the other hand, BALB/c mice presented a higher mortality rate (25%), but a later mean time of death (28,4 dpi) (**Figure 2C**). Since the same protocol and *T. cruzi* strain were used to infect both mouse lineages, we can suggest that the differences in the parasite load and mortality are influenced by immunological response developed by each mouse strain, which is determined by their genetic backgrounds. Nonetheless, the actual basis for that difference is unknown. BALB/c mice have been described to carry the susceptible genotype for the *Scl11c1* gene, a divalent ion transporter present on monocytes, macrophages, NK cells, and γδ T cells, which have roles in phagosome maturation, cell activation, and IFN production, rendering hosts susceptible to several intracellular pathogens, such as *Leishmania donovani*, *Salmonella typhimurium*, and *Mycobacterium sp* [54–56]. The A/J strain, on the other side, carries the resistant genotype [57, 58], being less susceptible to those pathogens. Nevertheless, this locus alone cannot explain host resistance to all pathogens, since BALB/c and A/J mice are both highly susceptible

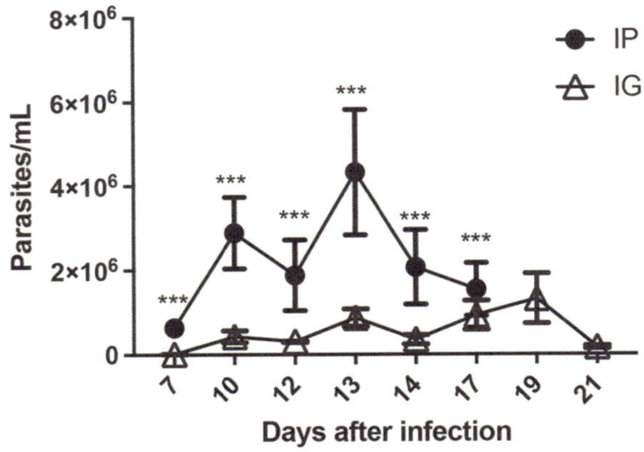


A

| Infection route | Infection rate | % of dead | Mean time to death |
|---|---|---|---|
| Intraperitoneal | 100% | 80% | 16,13 |
| Intragastric | 36% | 30% | 22,67 |

B

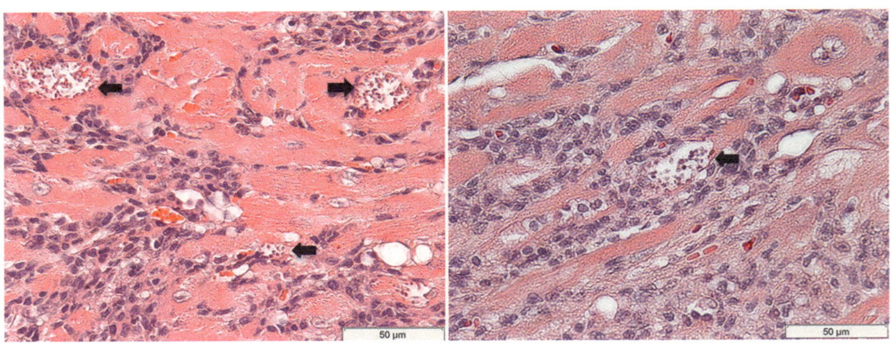


C D

**Figure 1.**
*Influence of the route of infection on parasitaemia, mortality, and heart histopathology. Swiss Webster outbred mice were infected either intraperitoneally (IP) or intragastrically (IG) with* $10^7$ *TCC of* Trypanosoma cruzi *SC2005 strain. Parasitaemia (A) shows an early and strong increase of parasites in the blood in IP-infected mice, which leads to an earlier time to death (B). IG-infected mice present a weak rate of infection (B) and a later and lighter parasitaemia (A). Nevertheless, both routes led to a colonization of the heart myocardium, which can be seen after 18 days on IP-infected mice (C) and 26 days on IG-infected animals (D). Hematoxylin and eosin. Arrows show parasite nests. Two-way ANOVA followed by Sidak's multiple comparison test.* *** = $p < 0.001$.

to *Staphylococcus aureus* infection [56] and BALB/c is resistant to hepatitis caused by Rift Valley Virus [57]. Susceptibility to infection is usually complex and dependent on multiple loci, which cannot be easily identified, but mouse genetics is a powerful tool to study host genetics.

In our study, BALB/c and A mice presented parasites nest on the heart (**Figure 2D** and **E**). Cardiac damage in acute Chagas disease is closely related to cases of death [5, 59]. The highest number of deaths observed in BALB/c *T. cruzi* SC2005-infected mice may be related to the extensive damage of the heart, caused not only by the parasite itself, but also to the inflammatory response against the parasite in this

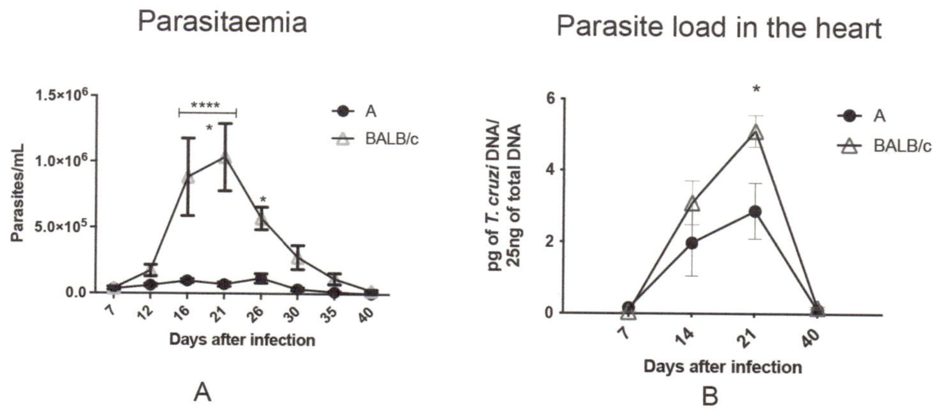


| Mouse background | % of dead | Mean time to death |
|---|---|---|
| A | 10% | 23,0 |
| BALB/c | 25% | 28,4 |

C

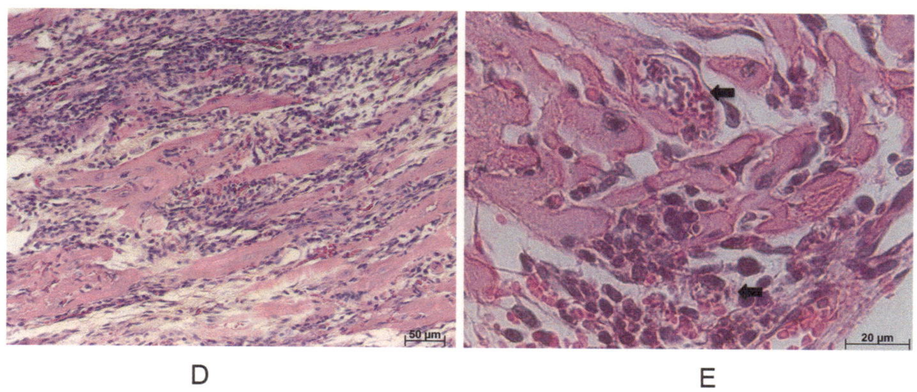


**Figure 2.**
*Influence of the mouse strain on the parasite load. Inbred mice from A and BALB/c genetic backgrounds were infected intragastrically (IG) with $10^7$ metacyclic forms of* Trypanosoma cruzi *SC2005 strain. BALB/c presented higher parasitaemia (A), higher parasite load on the heart, measured by qPCR (B) and higher mortality rate (C) than A mice. Histopathology from heart of BALB/c animals shows inflammatory infiltration (D) and parasite nests (E; arrows). Hematoxylin and eosin. Two-way ANOVA followed by Sidak's multiple comparison test. * = $p < 0.05$; **** = $p < 0.0001$.*

organ, once this mouse strain showed an inflammation on the heart more extensive and intense than A mice. A wide genomic association study carried out with patients from Colombia, Bolivia, and Argentina has identified a QTL in chromosome 11 which is associated with the development of Chagasic cardiomyopathy [28]. The QTL seems to correspond to a methylation site at the CCDC88B gene, which is involved in the inflammatory response [60].

### 3.2 *T. cruzi* SC2005 infection induces hematological alterations

In this work, hypochromic anemia was the main hematological alteration found after *T. cruzi* SC2005 intragastric infection. BALB/c mice showed hypochromic anemia earlier (14 dpi) than A-infected mice (21 dpi) (**Figure 3**). Anemia is a common hematological alteration observed in acute Chagas' disease, as described by Chagas in patients infected by *T. cruzi* [8]. In experimental infections, this hematological alteration also has been shown in different mouse strains [61]. However, the mechanisms responsible for this alteration are still unsolved. In acute *T. cruzi* infection, the lethality is associated with the reduced number of blood cells and the impaired bone marrow function [62]. All these alterations may be influenced by cytokine secretion and parasite or cell-dependent cytotoxicity in the blood and bone marrow [63].

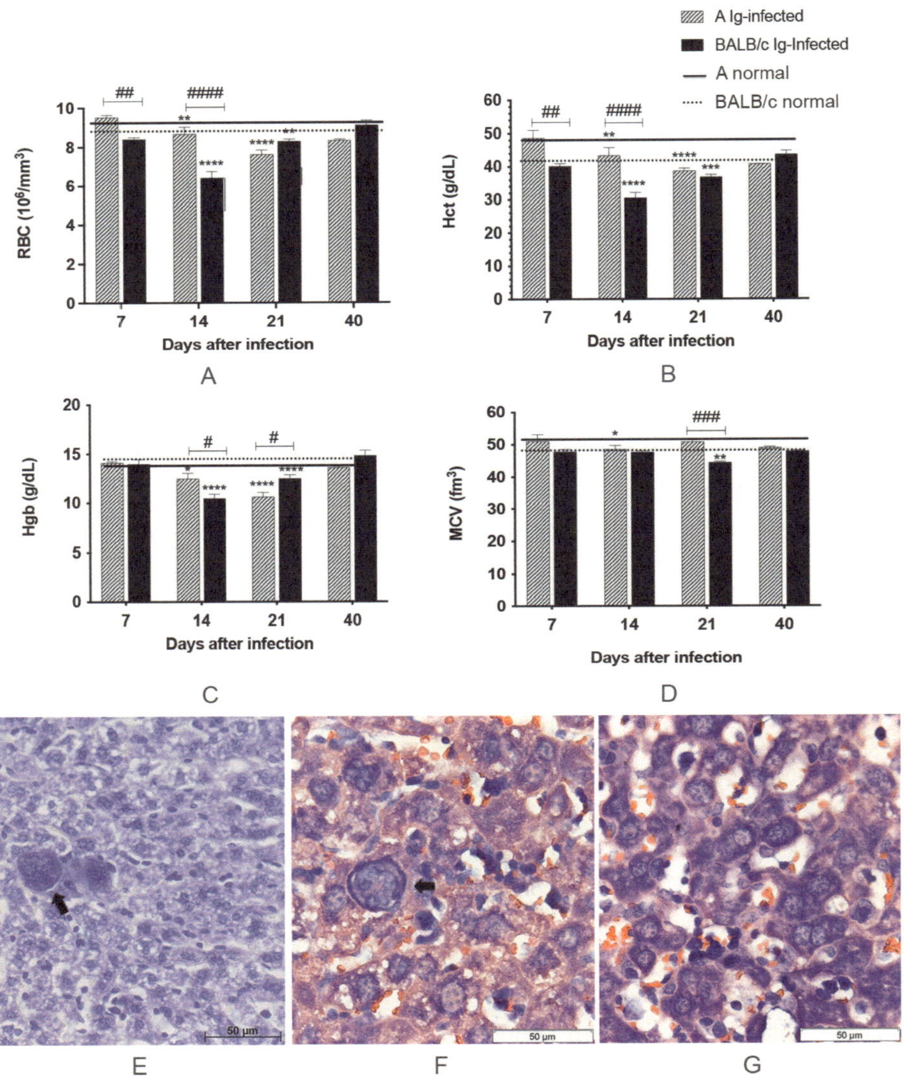


**Figure 3.**
*Hematological analysis. A-E inbred mice from A and BALB/c genetic backgrounds were infected intragastrically (Ig) with $10^7$ metacyclic forms of* Trypanosoma cruzi *SC2005 strain. BALB/c mice shows a reduction in red blood cells count (RBC; A), hematocrit (Hct; B), and hemoglubin (Hgb; C). The mean corpuscular volume (MCV) of BALB/c red blood cells also presented a slight reduction (D). Extracellular hematopoiesis could be observed in the liver of BALB/c mice (E) but also in outbred Swiss mice intraperitoneally infected with $10^7$ TCC of* T. cruzi *SC2005 strain (F), where immature cells are also observed (G). E: Giemsa; F and G: Hematoxylin and eosin. Two-way ANOVA followed by Sidak's multiple comparison test. * = $p < 0.05$; **p = <0.01; *** = $p < 0.001$; **** = $p < 0.0001$ in comparison with normal mice from the same background. # = $p < 0.05$; ## = $p < 0.01$; ### = $p < 0.001$; #### = $p < 0.0001$, comparing infected mice from different genetic backgrounds.*

A reduced life span or sequestration of RBC by autoantibodies or other mechanisms have been described as a factor that can contribute to anemia in protozoan and viral infections [64–69]. The average life span of a red blood cell is 40 days in a normal mouse [70]. In this study, *T. cruzi* infection reduced the life span of RBC contributing to anemia, once both mouse-infected strains showed an anemia earlier to this period, between 14 and 21 dpi (**Figure 3**).

Bone marrow suppression is related with the activity of several cytokines, and among them are TNF-α and IFN-γ [71–74]. It was shown that an excessive production of TNF-α and IFN-γ promotes damage in hematopoiesis in mice infected with lymphocytic choriomeningitis virus (LCMV) [71]. In studies with malaria, TNF-α has been described as an important anemia mediator [64]. In previous studies, inhibitory effects of TNF-α on erythropoiesis have been demonstrated [74, 75]. This inhibitory effect was also observed during acute infection by *T. cruzi*, in which the production of TNF-α by activated macrophages was correlated with a decrease in erythropoiesis [63]. In our study, the results indicate that the anemia observed after *T. cruzi* infection can be associated with a depressed bone marrow function induced by TNF-α and IFN-γ, once both infected mouse strains produced high levels of TNF-α and IFN-γ, 14 days after infection (see below), correlating with the decrease of RBC and Hgb (**Figure 3A** and **C**).

One consequence of the depressed bone marrow function, characterized by the poor quality or insufficiency of the blood elements production, is extramedullary hematopoiesis (EMH). EMH can occur in adult mouse livers [65, 66] under myelosuppression by various pathological lesions, including hemoglobinopathies, most commonly sickle cell anemia and thalassemia [67, 68]. In our study, we observed the occurrence of extramedullary hematopoiesis in the livers of *T. cruzi*-infected animals at 14 and 21 dpi, characterized by the presence of megakaryocytes, immature hematopoietic cells, and mitotic cells (**Figure 3E, F** and **G**). Altogether, these findings corroborate the hypothesis that *T. cruzi* SC2005 infection causing an impairment in bone marrow function, induced by TNF-α and IFN-γ, which lead to the occurrence of anemia and extramedullary hematopoiesis in mice livers as a compensatory mechanism.

Leukocytosis is another hematological alteration described after *T. cruzi* infection. A systematic review analyzing 31 articles up to 2016 showed that half of them described anemia in infected mammals and 68.2% described leukocytosis [76]. According to Tribullatti et al. [77], molecules such as chemokines, cytokines, antibodies, and nitric oxide produced during *T. cruzi* infection, together with molecules produced by the parasite itself, lead to hematological alterations in infected animals. In this study, a significant leukocytosis was observed in A and BALB/c mouse strains 21 and 40 days after *T. cruzi* SC2005 intragastric infection (**Figure 4A** and **B**). This leukocytosis was associated with the parasitemia levels and characterized by monocytosis and lymphocytosis, as well as by the presence of a lymphocytic atypia. When comparing infection routes, both IP- and IG-infected animals presented an increased number of leukocytes at the same time when parasitaemia increased. Nevertheless, leukocytosis is much higher in IG-infected mice ($p < 0.0001$, comparing leukocytosis peak, day 12 for IP- and 18 for IG-infected mice), even with a lower parasitaemia. In both cases, leukocytosis is caused mainly by an increase of lymphocytes, although neutrophils also follow the increase (**Figure 4C-F**). Several works previously reported alterations in leukocyte counts associated with parasitemia levels in different experimental models. Cynomolgus macaque (*Macaca fascicularis*) naturally infected by *T. cruzi* [78] and Rhesus monkeys experimentally infected with *T. cruzi* Colombian

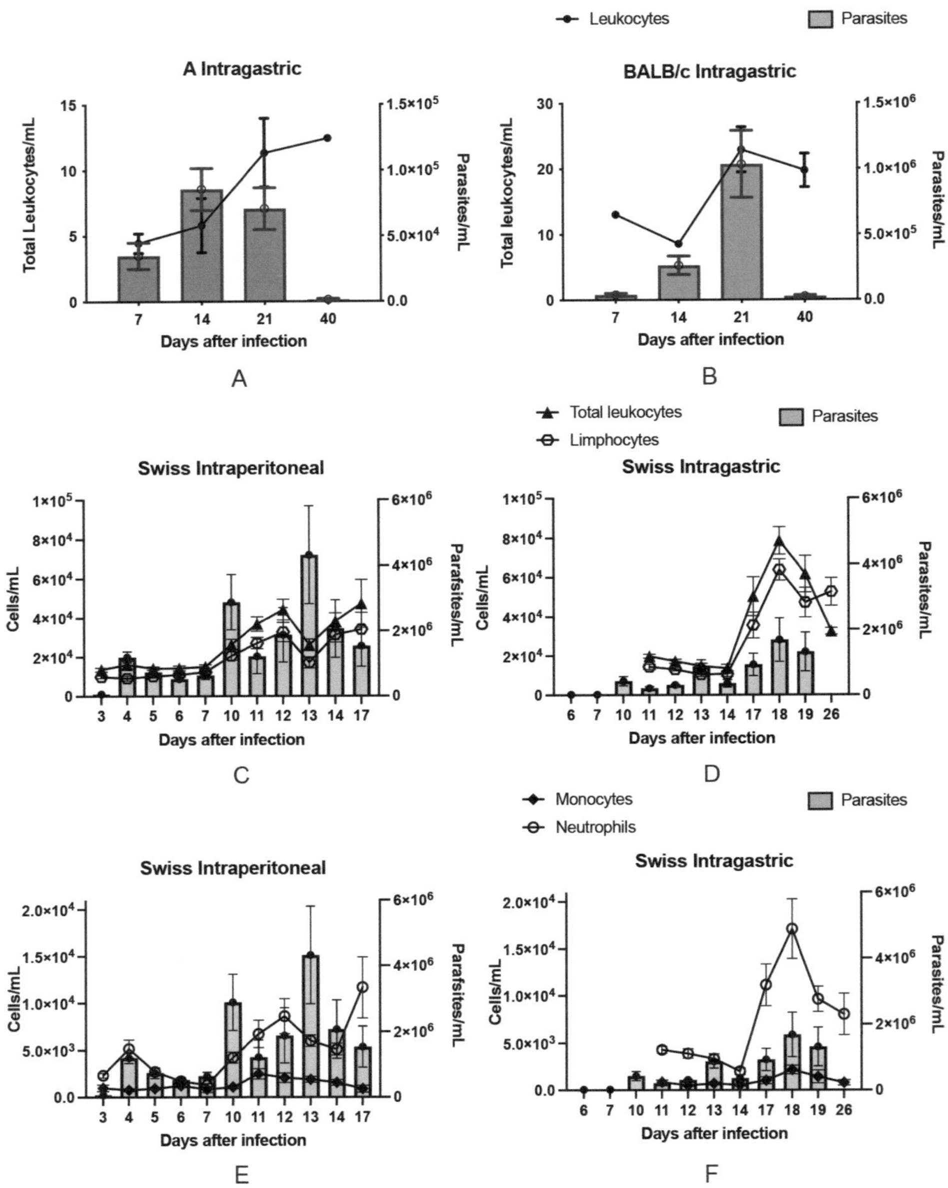


**Figure 4.**
*White blood cell count analysis. Inbred mice from A (A) and BALB/c (B) genetic backgrounds intragastrically infected with $10^7$ metacyclic forms of* Trypanosoma cruzi *SC2005 strain presented leukocytosis associated with parasitaemia. C-F. Swiss Webster outbred mice were infected either intraperitoneally or intragastrically with $10^7$ TCC of* T. cruzi *SC2005 strain. Mice infected intragastrically show an increase in the total leukocytes, lymphocytes (D), and neutrophils (F) at the same time of the parasitemic peak.*

strain [79] showed a positive correlation between leukocytosis, lymphocytosis, and parasitemia peaks. The same correlation was found in Beagle dogs infected by different *T. cruzi* strains [80, 81]. On the other hand, other authors obtained the contradictory results during experimental murine infection with *T. cruzi* CL strain in C3H mice, showing an exponential growth of parasites accompanied by leukopenia in these animals [82]. Such dissimilarity in experimental data suggests that both the host

DOI: http://dx.doi.org/10.5772/intechopen.104461

genetic background and the *T. cruzi* strain may influence the hematological alterations occurring after infection.

### 3.3 Immune response in *T. cruzi* SC2005-infected mice

Recognition of *T. cruzi* by macrophages and dendritic cells leads to phagocytosis and elicits a predominately T helper type 1 (Th1) response with the production of pro-inflammatory cytokines (i.e., IFN-γ, IL-2, IL-6, IL-12, and TNF-α) [83–85]. This promotes an antiparasitic response, with differentiation and proliferation of Th1 CD4+ cells, activation of CD8+ T cells, and macrophages [86]. The recognition of *T. cruzi*-infected cells and effective control of infection during the acute and chronic phases are mainly related to the action of effector CD8+ T cells [48, 79, 87]. More severe clinical disease is associated with reduced CD8+ T cell responses and the boost of CD8+ T cell response after treatment improves the clinical outcome [88, 89]. However, studies indicate that, in the absence of $CD4^+$ T cells, $CD8^+$ T lymphocytes fail to restrain the parasite growth [90], because $CD4^+$ T lymphocytes are responsible for promoting the macrophages activation and $CD8^+$ T and B cells proliferation. Therefore, its deficiency leads to an overall reduction of host immune response and a consequent increase in tissue parasitism [91].

In our study, the frequencies of $CD4^+$, $CD8^+$, $CD4^+/CD8^+$ T cells and B cells in different organs varied according to the route of infection, and mouse strain. After intraperitoneal infection by *T. cruzi* SC2005 strain, Swiss mice presented an increase in $CD4^+$ T cells frequency in the spleen at 18 dpi. On the other hand, IG-infected mice showed an increase in the frequencies of $CD8^+$ T cells 26 and 33 dpi (**Figure 5A**). The increase of these cells corroborates with the increase in spleen weight (**Figure 6A**), caused by the intense production of cells, as shown by the hyperplasia of the germinal center induced by both infection routes in this organ (**Figure 6B** and **C**). An increase in the cellularity and size of spleen, caused by the amplification of T and B lymphocytes polyclonal activation, has been previously described during *T. cruzi* infection [92].

In the blood, IG-infected mice showed a reduction of $CD4^+$ T cells frequency (26 dpi) and an increase of $CD8^+$ T cells 26 and 33 days after infection (**Figure 5B**). Meanwhile, the analysis of lymph nodes showed a decrease of $CD4^+$ T cell frequency on both infected groups: IP-infected mice at 11 dpi and IG-infected mice 26 and 33 dpi (**Figure 5C**). The variation in the T cells frequency in the mesenteric lymph nodes is caused by depletion of lymphocytes and increased apoptosis rates, which may be related to the production of different cytokines [92].

These results show a fluctuation in the percentage of lymphocytes in the analyzed tissues. This variation demonstrates the differentiated role of each compartment and a different response profile with a specific and coordinated response of these sites against the parasite [93]. Besides, we demonstrated the influence of infection route on the lymphocyte's frequency and magnitude, once *T. cruzi* IG-infected mice showed a higher expansion of $CD8^+$ T cells in the spleen and blood.

The differences in expansion and distribution of T and B cell frequencies in the blood, liver, and heart of A and BALB/c mice IG infected by *T. cruzi* SC2005 were also demonstrated in this work. SC2005 *T. cruzi* IG infection induced an increase of $CD8^+$ T and $CD4^+/CD8^+$ T lymphocytes in all analyzed organs on both mouse strains, although in A mice the increase occurred earlier than in BALB/c mice. The infection also induced a decrease in $CD4^+$ T cell and B lymphocyte frequencies in the heart and blood of infected animals (**Figure 7**). It is known that in both acute and chronic

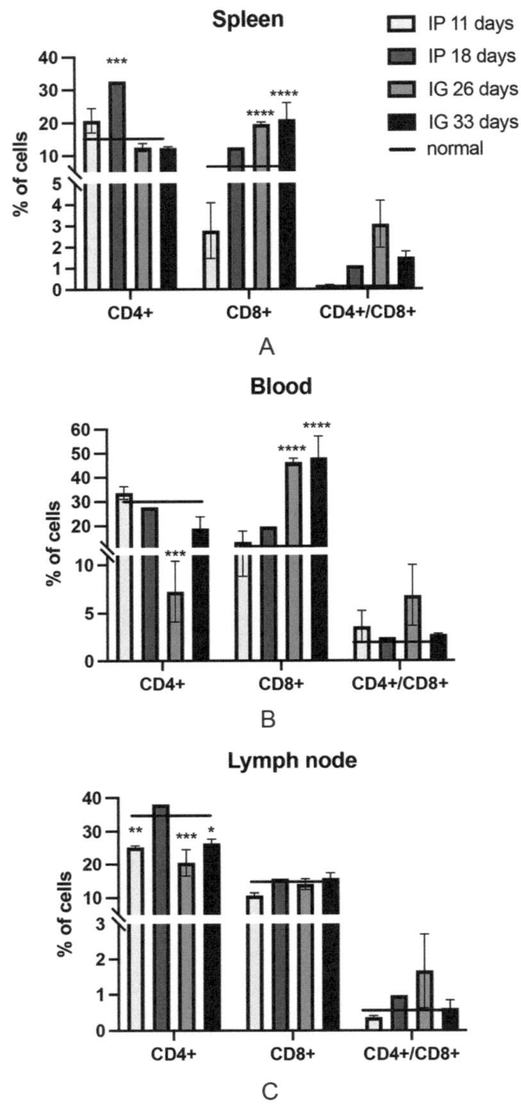


**Figure 5.**
*T cells present in the inflammatory infiltrate. Swiss Webster outbred mice were infected either intraperitoneally (IP) or intragastrically (IG) with $10^7$ TCC of* Trypanosoma cruzi *SC2005 strain. Intragastrically-infected mice show an increase of T CD8$^+$ cells in the spleen (A) and blood (B), but not in the draining lymph node (C). IP = intraperitoneally infected; IG = intragastrically infected. Two-way ANOVA followed by Sidak's multiple comparison test, in comparison to non-infected normal mice.* * = $p < 0.05$; *** = $p < 0.001$; **** = $p < 0.0001$.

*T. cruzi* infections, the increase of CD8$^+$ T lymphocytes is common [69]. Increased levels of these cells have been described as Chagas disease biomarkers in humans and monkeys naturally infected by *T. cruzi* [70]. CD8$^+$ T cell type-1 (Tc1) subsets are the main cause of *T. cruzi* death through the production of both IFN-γ and TNF-α [94, 95], contributing to the control of parasitaemia levels [91, 96, 97]. In this study, BALB/c and A mice infected by *T. cruzi* SC2005 presented lymphocytosis (**Figure 4A** and **B**) and an increase of CD8$^+$ T cells in the blood at the same time of the parasitaemia peak (21 dpi), remaining until the end of the experiment (40 dpi), when the parasite load was very low (**Figure 2A**). These results reinforce the previous

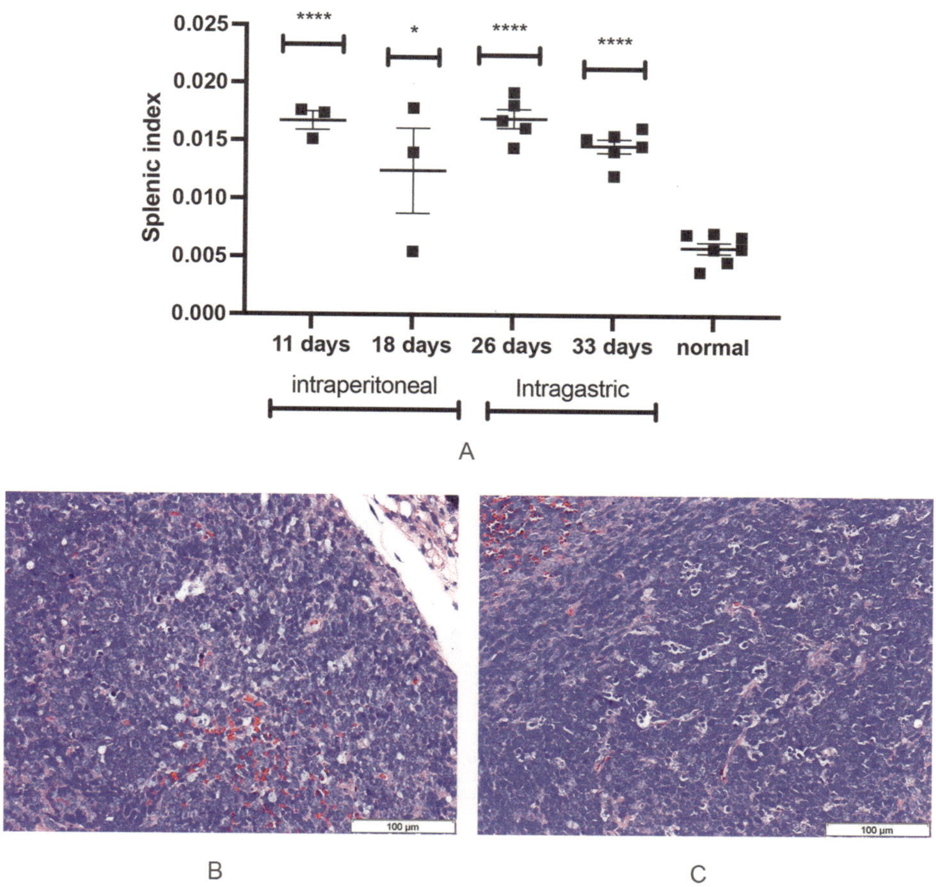


**Figure 6.**
*Cell proliferation in the spleen. Swiss Webster outbred mice were infected either intraperitoneally or intragastrically with $10^7$ TCC of* Trypanosoma cruzi *SC2005 strain. All mice present a higher spleen index (A) than normal mice, showing cell proliferation is occurring on the organ, which is corroborated with histopathology image from intraperitoneally (B) and intragastrically (C) infected mice. Hematoxylin and eosin. One-way ANOVA followed by Sidak's multiple comparison test.* * $= p < 0.05$; **** $= p < 0.0001$.

observations about the role of $CD8^+$ T cells in the control of parasitaemia levels and its probable cytotoxic activity against the parasite, as reported previously [78].

$CD4^+/CD8^+$ double-positive T cells, under normal conditions, are found in the thymus, where they undergo differentiation into mature $CD4^+$ and $CD8^+$ T cells. During *T. cruzi* infection, there is a significant impairment of this organ, due to a deregulated cascade of proinflammatory cytokines. This impairment leads to cell maturation in extrathymic organs such as the bone marrow and liver [98, 99]. In this study, the increase of the $CD4^+/CD8^+$ T double-positive cells frequency in the heart, liver, and blood indicates an impairment of the thymus and consequent liberation of immature cells in the circulation or the occurrence of extracellular hematopoiesis in the liver (**Figure 3E**).

In *T. cruzi* infection, the clearance of blood trypomastigotes occurs in the liver [100], regardless of the gateway. The liver is the main organ involved in the defense against disseminating blood pathogens, being critical to host immunity and survival [101, 102]. In this work, an increase of both $CD8^+$ T cells and $CD19^+$ B cells was observed in the hepatic parenchyma (**Figure 7C**). B cells act as antigen-presenting

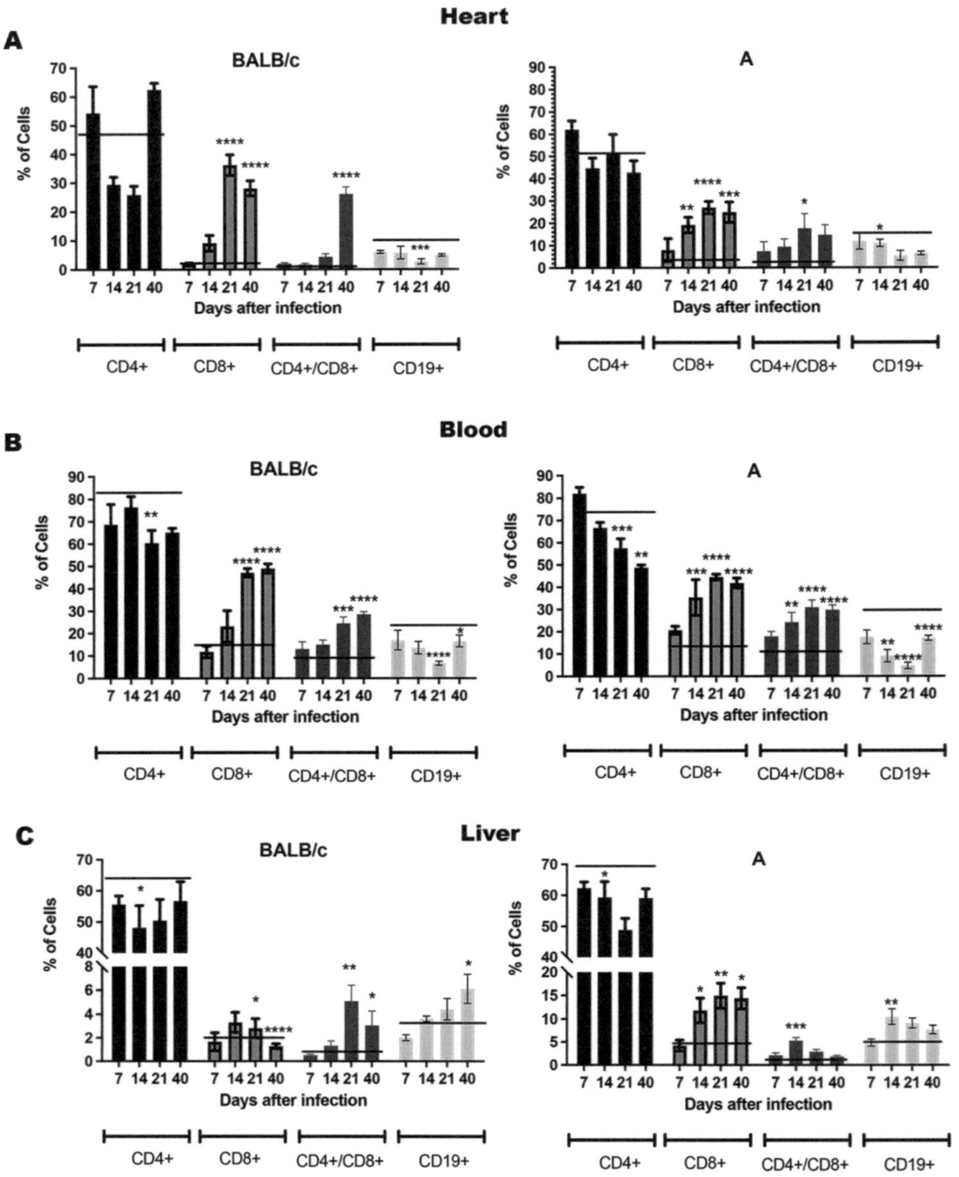


**Figure 7.**
*Influence of the mouse strain on cell recruitment. Inbred mice from A and BALB/c genetic backgrounds were infected intragastrically (IG) with $10^7$ metacyclic forms of* Trypanosoma cruzi *SC2005 strain.* T. cruzi *Infection caused an increase of CD8+ cells on the heart (A), blood (B) and liver (C) of infected mice. However, BALB/c CD8+ cells increased from 21 days after infection, whereas at 14 days after infection A mice already presented higher frequencies of CD8+ cells. The same happened with CD4+/CD8+ in mice blood. (B) CD19+ cell frequency was reduced in the blood from both mouse strains. Lines show normal mice mean frequencies. Two-way ANOVA followed by Sidak's multiple comparison test in comparison with normal mice from the same background.*
$^{*} = p < 0.05$; $^{**} = p < 0.01$; $^{***} = p < 0.001$; $^{****} = p < 0.0001$.

cells (APC), in the secretion of antibodies, and in the activation of $CD8^+$ T cells [103]. Besides, they have been implicated in the mobilization of inflammatory cells to the tissues and are fundamental to the control of parasite growth, by triggering a Th1 response [90, 104, 105]. The observation of these cells in the liver suggests the role of $CD19^+$ cells as antigen-present cells (APC). A mice showed an earlier increase of these cell frequencies (14 dpi) than BALB/c-infected mice (21 dpi) (**Figure 7C**). The early presence of B and CD8$^+$ T cells in the liver of A mice indicates the importance of this organ in parasite clearance and may explain why this mouse strain has lower parasite load and mortality.

Redistribution and circulation of lymphocyte subtypes to other sites are modulated by the local and systemic immune system [106]. This regulation is affected by the infection and often related to the severity of the clinical manifestations.

Several murine studies have described the importance of proinflammatory cytokines during *T. cruzi* infection. C57BL/6 IL-17A knockout (IL-17A −/−) mice infected by *T. cruzi* Tulahuén strain showed a reduced production of IFN-γ, IL-6, and TNF-α cytokines, which was related to a more severe parasitemia and mortality, than observed in wild-type mice [107]. On the other hand, an improvement of the mice resistance to parasite growth was observed when IL-18 or 5-lipoxygenase was inhibited, generating an increase in the IL-12, IFN-γ, IL-1β, and IL-6 levels during the acute phase of disease [108, 109]. Studies *in vitro*, using PBMC infected by *T. cruzi* Tulahuén strain, indicate that IL-6 improves the survival and effector functions of cytotoxic cells [110]. These data reveal the important role of these cytokines in the control of *T. cruzi* infection and host mortality. In the present work, both infected mouse strains produced a similar pattern of TNF-α, IFN-γ, and IL-6 production, but A-infected mice showed an earlier increase in the production of these cytokines, when compared to BALB/c mice (**Figure 8**).

### 3.4 Histopathological alterations caused by SC2005 *T. cruzi* infection

After infection, *T. cruzi* can be detected in several organs/tissues and induce an inflammatory response, which can be found even where the parasite is not detected [111, 112]. The preferential tropism, as well as distinct local and systemic immune responses can be influenced by different transmission routes of *T. cruzi* [39, 47, 112, 113] as well as by the host genetic background [114].

In this study, we observed differences in the parasite load and inflammatory infiltrate intensity depending on the inoculation route used. IP infection showed an higher tissue colonization by SC2005 *T. cruzi* and a more intense inflammatory infiltrate than in IG infection. IP-infected mice showed a moderate-to-intense diffuse mononuclear inflammatory infiltrate (composed mainly by monocytes and lymphocytes) in the esophagus, stomach, intestine, heart, liver, pancreas, adrenal gland, bladder, uterus, trachea, and adipose tissue (**Figure 9**). Parasite nests were observed in the stomach (**Figure 9A**), esophagus (**Figure 9B**), intestine, heart, pancreas, bladder, and adipose tissue. Mast cells were observed only at 18 dpi in inflammatory infiltrates of the heart, stomach, and adipose tissue (**Figure 9D**). Severe pancreatitis with focal necrosis were also observed (**Figure 9E** and **F**) and the liver of the infected mice showed immature cells, megakaryocytes, and dividing cells (**Figure 3F** and **G**). In addition, a redistribution and increase of collagen fibers, associated with inflammatory infiltrates, was observed in the esophagus, heart (**Figure 9G**), stomach (**Figure 9H**), bladder, and uterus. Thymus and brain showed no changes in these animals.

On the other hand, IG infection induced a moderate-to-intense diffuse inflammatory infiltrate essentially lymphomonocytic in the esophagus, stomach, liver, kidney, bladder, uterus, brain, intestine, heart, pancreas, and adipose tissue (**Figure 10**). Mast cells were observed in the inflammatory infiltrates of the adipose tissue, bladder, and stomach (**Figure 10A**). Parasite nests were observed in lower numbers than IP-infected mice only in stomach, heart, bladder (**Figure 10D**), and adipose tissue. Thymus

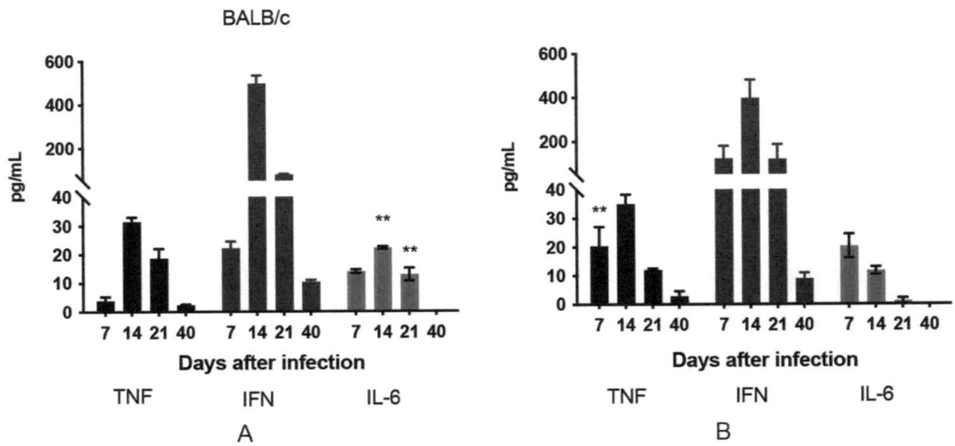


**Figure 8.**
*Cytokine production by mice from different strains. Inbred mice from BALB/c (A) and A (B) genetic backgrounds were infected intragastrically (IG) with $10^7$ metacyclic forms of* Trypanosoma cruzi *SC2005 strain. Both strain presented similar cytokine production, although it starts earlier in A mice. Two-way ANOVA followed by Sidak's multiple comparison test. ## = $p < 0.01$, in comparison with the other mouse strain.*

showed no changes in these animals. A common alteration observed in both IP- and IG-infected animals was the germinal centers hyperplasia in spleen and lymph nodes (**Figure 6C**), as well as omental and mesenteric milky spots were activated (**Figure 10C**), and myeloid cells are present. In addition, the liver of the infected mice showed immature cells, megakaryocytes, and dividing cells.

Both infected mice showed a redistribution and an increase of collagen fibers, associated with inflammatory infiltrates and a decrease of these infiltrates with the course of infection, with exception of the heart, where there is an increase of these infiltrates in the later times (IP-18 dpi and IG-33 dpi). These inflammatory infiltrates were preferentially located in the muscle layer of the organs. In the heart, they were preferentially located in the atria, while parasites were found in the heart ventricles. IP-infected mice showed an increase in heart parasitism at 18 dpi. On the contrary, IG-infected mice showed scarce parasite nests in this organ at 33 dpi and a much larger inflammatory infiltrate (essentially lymphoid) than observed in IP-infected mice (**Figure 1C** and **D**).

Similar to the observed Swiss mice infected by IG or IP routes, A and BALB/c mice IG infected by SC2005 *T. cruzi* strain showed immature cells and megakaryocytes in the liver (**Figure 3E**); and mononuclear inflammatory infiltrates associated with the increase of collagen fibers in several tissues (**Figure 11**). Both mouse strains presented inflammatory infiltrates in several organs, but in BALB/c the stomach (21 and 40 dpi), heart (14 and 21 dpi) (**Figure 2D**), and liver (7 dpi) were more inflamed. On the other hand, the esophagus of A mice presented an intense inflammatory infiltrate, whereas BALB/c's did not show any alterations. Neither mouse strains present histopathological changes in the gut (**Figure 11A**).

As it can be observed, the SC2005 *T. cruzi* infection induced similar alterations independent of the route of infection (IP or IG) and the mouse strain (BALB/c or A). The histopathological analysis showed a mononuclear infiltrate mainly located in the muscular layers, which was associated with neoformation and remodeling of collagen fibers in different organs (**Figure 11D** and **E**). Studies with *T. cruzi* strains

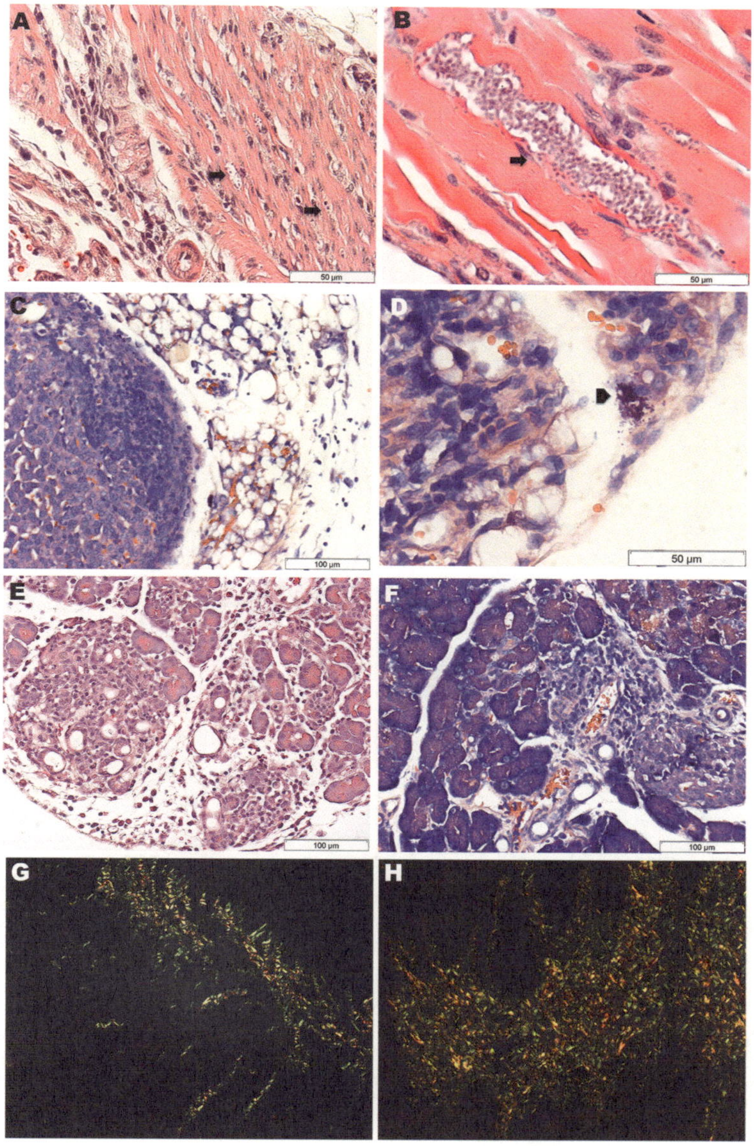


**Figure 9.**
*Histopathological alterations in intragastrically-infected mice. Swiss Webster outbred mice were intraperitoneally (IP) infected with $10^7$ TCC of* Trypanosoma cruzi *SC2005 strain. Inflammatory infiltration and parasite nests (arrows) can be observed in mice stomach (A) and esophagus (B). Different other tissues also present intense inflammation, including supra renal (C) and adipocytes, in which we can observe mast cells (arrow head) (D). IP infected mice presented severe pancreatite (E and F). Collagen fibers can be observed in heart (G) and stomach (H) of mice. Hematoxylin and eosin (A-F) and Picrus Sirius red in polarized light (G-H).*

belonging to the biodemes type II and III showed the same histopathological patterns of localization of inflammatory infiltration [5]. The deposition of collagen and the tissue remodeling during *T. cruzi* infection have already been described in several studies [115–117]. In the heart, amastigote nests were present more frequently in the ventricles than in the atria. However, the atria presented a more intense inflammatory infiltration than ventricles. These findings suggest that the inflammatory

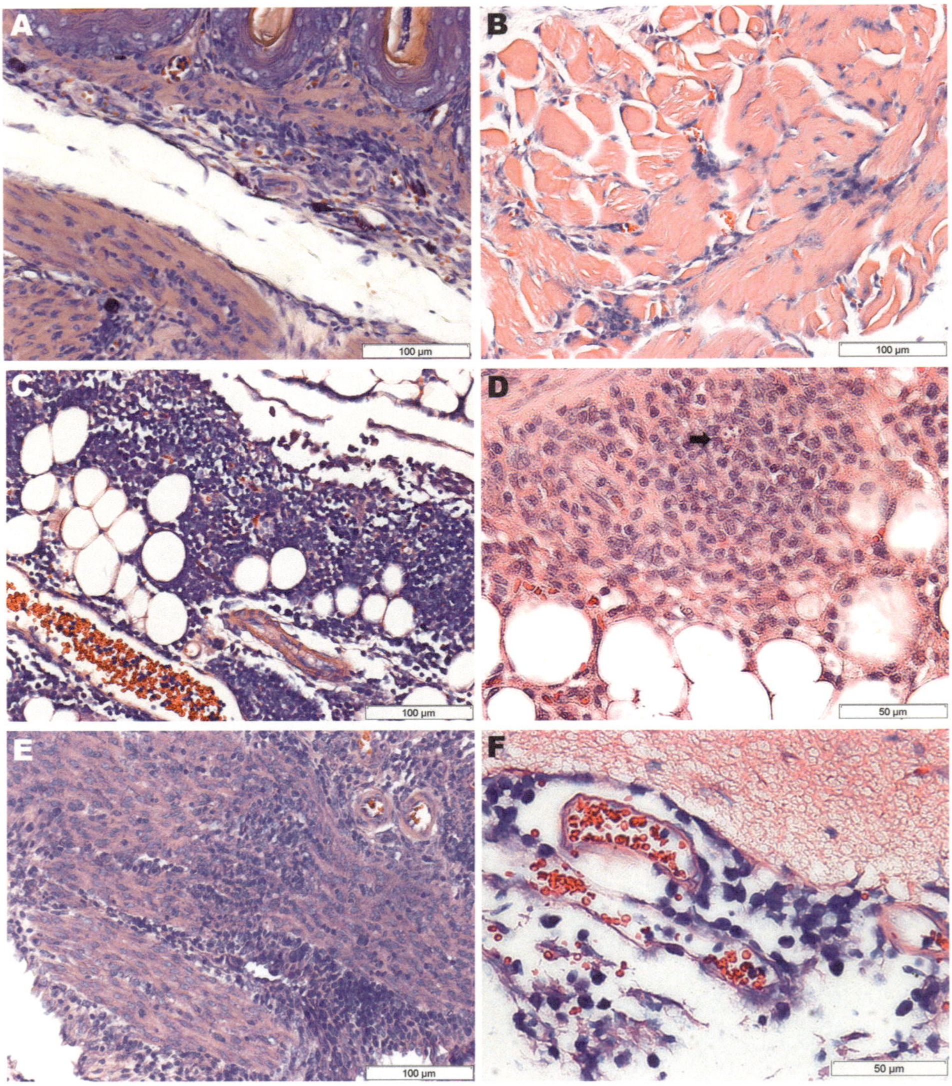


**Figure 10.**
*Histopathological alterations in intraperitoneal infected mice. Swiss Webster outbred mice were intragastrically (IG) infected with* $10^7$ *TCC of* Trypanosoma cruzi *SC2005 strain. Moderate inflammatory infiltrate are present in different tissues such as stomach (A), esophagus (B), intestine (C), bladder (D), uterus (E), and meninges (F). Several mast cells can be observed in mice stomach (A). Activated milk spots are present in the intestine (C) and small parasite nests were observed in the bladder (arrow) (D). Hematoxylin and eosin.*

response against the parasite first occurs in the auricular tissue and only later reaches the ventricular tissue. It is interesting to note that Quijano-Hernández et al. in 2012 [118] observed the same histopathological patterns in infected dogs. Cardiac damages are closely related to cases of death in acute Chagas disease [5, 59]. In this study, a larger cardiac involvement and a higher parasite load were observed in the hearts of BALB/c-infected mice. The extensive damage of the heart plus the large number of parasite DNA and a late $CD8^+$ T cell response, corroborate to the highest number of deaths in this group.

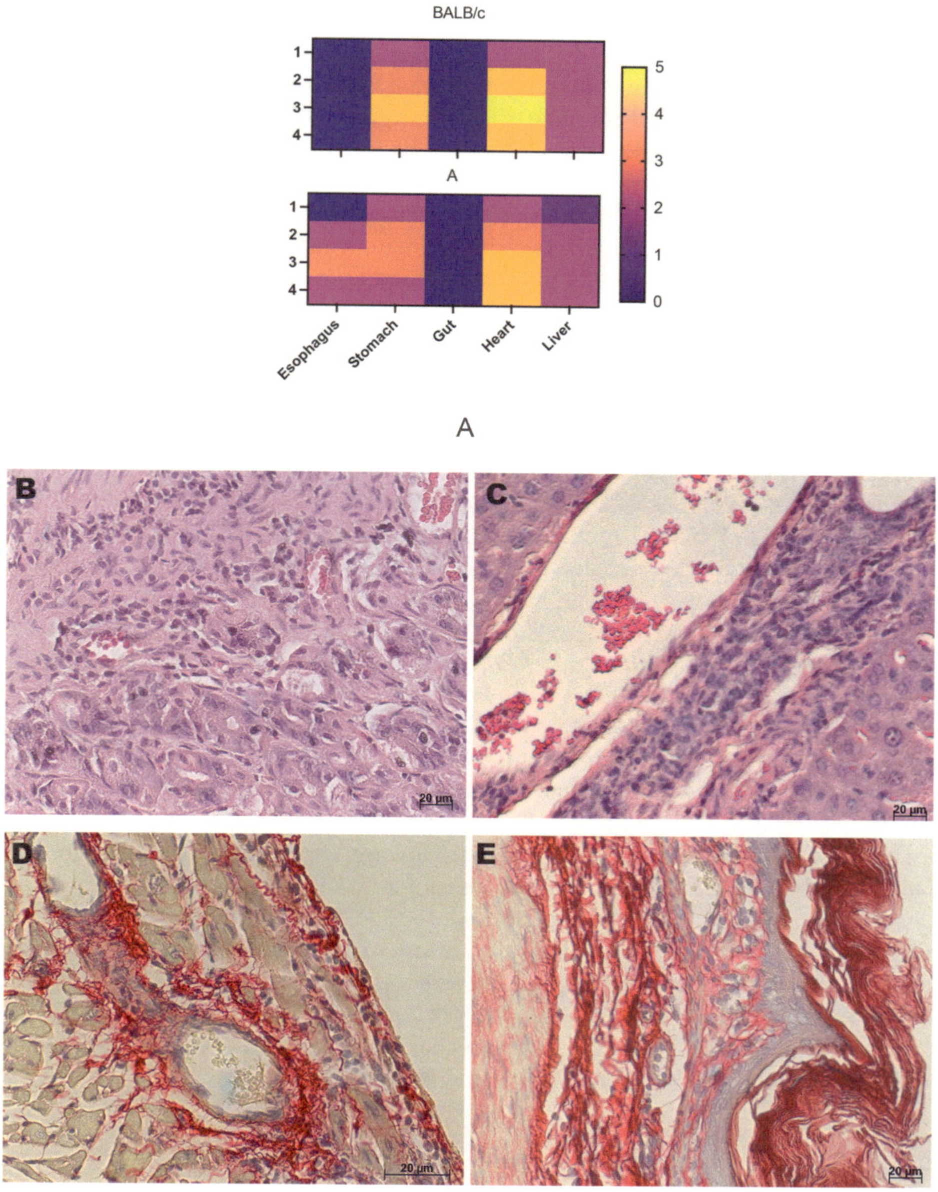


**Figure 11.**
*Histopathological alterations in intragastrically-infected BALB/c mice. Inbred BALB/c mice were infected intragastrically (IG) with $10^7$ metacyclic forms of* Trypanosoma cruzi *SC2005 strain. Inflammatory infiltration was quantified in various organs (A) inflammation can be observed in mice stomach (B) and liver (C). Alteration of collagen fibers are also observed in heart (D), and stomach (E). Hematoxylin and eosin (B-C) and Picrus Sirius red (D-E).*

The presence of immature cells and megakaryocytes in the liver was also a common finding in all infected mice. This finding suggests that extramedullary hematopoiesis was occurring in this organ. During the acute phase of *T. cruzi* infection, Marcondes et al. in 2000 [82] demonstrated alterations in blood cell counts associated with bone marrow suppression and anemia, which explain the occurrence of extramedullary hematopoiesis.

## 4. Conclusion

Altogether, the findings of this study point that *T. cruzi* SC2005 strain can spread through the bloodstream and colonize different organs and tissues, producing a systemic response, which is variable depending on the inoculation route and the genetic background of the host. Heart and stomach were the most intensely parasitized and inflamed organs in all models. *T. cruzi* SC2005 strain infects preferentially the muscular layers of the organs, where inflammatory infiltrates are also observed with higher intensity, being associated with an increase and redistribution of collagen fibers. In the heart, inflammatory infiltrates are preferentially located in the atria, while parasites are mostly found in the ventricles.

*T. cruzi* SC2005 intragastric infection induces a hypochromic anemia, and an extramedullary hematopoiesis in mouse livers, characterized by the presence of immature cells and megakaryocytes, as well as an increase of $CD4^+/CD8^+$ frequencies, corroborating the hypothesis that *T. cruzi* SC2005 infection causes an impairment in bone marrow function. Besides, the infection also induces a leukocytosis, characterized by an increase of $CD8^+$ T lymphocytes, as well as an increase of proinflammatory cytokines production. The increase of leukocytes was correlated with the increase of parasitaemia.

The intraperitoneal infection proved to be more infective and severe than the intragastric route, leading to a higher parasitaemia, mortality, tissue colonization, and tissue inflammatory response.

The mouse strain influences the immune response, pointing to a role for host genetics in the susceptibility to infection. In this study, although *T. cruzi* SC2005 intragastric infection has been induced a similar profile of changes in A and BALB/c mice, the earlier development of a proinflammatory cytotoxic cellular profile of A mice led to a less severe disease outcome, with lower parasite load and mortality. Infected A mice also exhibited an early induction of $CD8^+$ T cells and proinflammatory cytokine production. On the other hand, for BALB/c-infected mice the response to infection occurred later, after a considerable increase in parasitemia, favoring the parasite multiplication and spread, and consequent higher mortality rate and tissue inflammation.

This study adds highlights on the factors that influence the pathology of Chagas disease, helping in the understanding of its different outcomes.

## Acknowledgements

The authors would like to thank the Flow Cytometry Core Facilities of the Instituto Oswaldo Cruz/FIOCRUZ-RJ. We also thank Sandy Santos Pereira for providing technical support, and Thaize Q. Chometon for operating the Cytoflex Flow Cytometer.

This work was supported by CAPES by student scholarship and Oswaldo Cruz Institute.

## Conflict of interest

The authors declare no conflict of interest.

## Author details

Flávia de Oliveira Cardoso*, Carolina Salles Domingues, Tânia Zaverucha do Valle and Kátia da Silva Calabrese
Laboratório de Imunomodulação e Protozoologia, Instituto Oswaldo Cruz, Fundação Oswaldo Cruz, Rio de Janeiro, Brazil

*Address all correspondence to: flaviaoc@ioc.fiocruz.br

## References

[1] WHO. Chagas Disease (Also Known as American Trypanosomiasis). WHO; 2021 Accessed: January 22, 2022. Available from: https://www.who.int/news-room/fact-sheets/detail/chagas-disease-(American-trypanosomiasis)

[2] Molyneux DH, Savioli L, Engels D. Neglected tropical diseases: Progress towards addressing the chronic pandemic. The Lancet. 2017;**389**:312-325

[3] Gascon J, Bern C, Pinazo MJ. Chagas disease in Spain, the United States and other non-endemic countries. Acta Tropica. Jul 2010;**115**(1-2):22-27

[4] World Health Organization. Global Distribution of Cases of Chagas Disease, Based on Official Estimates, 2018. Accessed: August 6, 2020. Available from: https://www.who.int/docs/default-source/ntds/chagas-disease/chagas-2018-cases.pdf?sfvrsn=f4e94b3b_2

[5] Zingales B, Miles MA, Campbell DA, Tibayrenc M, Macedo AM, Teixeira MMG, et al. The revised *Trypanosoma cruzi* subspecific nomenclature: Rationale, epidemiological relevance and research applications. Infection, Genetics and Evolution. 2012;**12**(2):240-253. DOI: 10.1016/j.meegid.2011.12.009

[6] Zingales B. *Trypanosoma cruzi* genetic diversity: Something new for something known about Chagas disease manifestations, serodiagnosis and drug sensitivity. Acta Tropica. 2018;**184**:38-52. DOI: 10.1016/j.actatropica.2017.09.017

[7] Lima L, Espinosa-Álvarez O, Ortiz PA, Trejo-Varón JA, Carranza JC, Pinto CM, et al. Genetic diversity of *Trypanosoma cruzi* in bats, and multilocus phylogenetic and phylogeographical analyses supporting Tcbat as an independent DTU (discrete typing unit). Acta Tropica. 2015;**151**(1):166-177

[8] Chagas C. Nova tripanosomiaze humana. Memórias do Instituto Oswaldo Cruz. 1909;**1**:3-62

[9] Angheben A, Boix L, Buonfrate D, Gobbi F, Bisoffi Z, Pupella S, et al. Chagas disease and transfusion medicine: A perspective from non-endemic countries. Blood Transfusion. 2015;**13**(4):540-550

[10] Schmuñis GA. Chagas' disease and blood transfusion. Progress in Clinical and Biological Research. 1985;**182**:127-145

[11] Sánchez LV, Ramírez JD. Congenital and oral transmission of American trypanosomiasis: An overview of physiopathogenic aspects. Parasitology. 2013;**140**(2):147-159

[12] Dias JCP, Neto VA. Prevention concerning the different alternative routes for transmission of *Trypanosoma cruzi* in Brazil. Revista da Sociedade Brasileira de Medicina Tropical. 2011;**44**(3):68-72

[13] Salvador F, Sánchez-Montalvá A, Sulleiro E, Moreso F, Berastegui C, Caralt M, et al. Prevalence of chagas disease among solid organ-transplanted patients in a nonendemic country. American Journal of Tropical Medicine and Hygiene. 2018;**98**(3):742-746

[14] Radisic MV, Repetto SA. American trypanosomiasis (Chagas disease) in solid organ transplantation. Transplant Infectious Disease. 2020;**22**(6):e13429

[15] Herwaldt BL. Laboratory-acquired parasitic infections from accidental exposures. Clinical Microbiology Reviews. 2001;**14**(4):659-688

[16] Araujo PF, Almeida AB, Pimentel CF, da Silva AR, Sousa A, Valente SA, et al. Sexual transmission of American trypanosomiasis in humans: A new potential pandemic route for chagas parasites. Memorias do Instituto Oswaldo Cruz. 2017;**112**(6):437-446

[17] Filigheddu MT, Górgolas M, Ramos JM. Orally-transmitted Chagas disease. Medicina Clinica. 2017;**148**(3): 125-131

[18] Alberto Toso M, Felipe Vial U, Galanti N. Transmisión de la enfermedad de Chagas por vía oral. Revista Medica de Chile. 2011;**139**(2):258-266

[19] Shikanai-Yasuda MA, Carvalho NB. Oral transmission of chagas disease. Clinical Infectious Diseases. 2012;**54**(6): 845-852

[20] Lidani KCF, Andrade FA, Bavia L, Damasceno FS, Beltrame MH, Messias-Reason IJ, et al. Chagas disease: From discovery to a worldwide health problem. Frontiers in Public Health. 2019;**7**:166

[21] Rueda K, Trujillo JE, Carranza JC, Vallejo GA. Transmisión oral de *Trypanosoma cruzi*: una nueva situación epidemiológica de la enfermedad de Chagas en Colombia y otros países suramericanos. Biomédica. 2014;**34**(4):631-641

[22] Macedo AM, Machado CR, Oliveira RP, SDJ P. *Trypanosoma cruzi*: Genetic structure of populations and relevance of genetic variability to the pathogenesis of chagas disease. Fundacao Oswaldo Cruz. 2004;**99**, Memorias do Instituto Oswaldo Cruz:1-12

[23] Campbell D, Westenberger S, Sturm N. The determinants of Chagas disease: Connecting parasite and host genetics. Current Molecular Medicine. 2004;**4**(6):549-562. Available from: https://pubmed.ncbi.nlm.nih.gov/15357207/

[24] Lewis MD, Francisco AF, Jayawardhana S, Langston H, Taylor MC, Kelly JM. Imaging the development of chronic Chagas disease after oral transmission. Scientific Reports. 2018;**8**(1):11292

[25] Souza W. O parasita e sua interação com os hospedeiros. In: Brenner Z, Andrade ZA, Barral-Neto M, editors. *Trypanosoma cruzi* e doença de Chagas. Rio de Janeiro: Guanabara Koogan; 1999. pp. 126-188

[26] Martinez SJ, Romano PS, Engman DM. Precision health for Chagas disease: Integrating parasite and host factors to predict outcome of infection and response to therapy. Frontiers in Cellular and Infection Microbiology. 2020;**8**(10):210

[27] Acosta-Herrera M, Strauss M, Casares-Marfil D, Martín J. Genomic medicine in Chagas disease. Acta Tropica. 2019;**1**(197):105062

[28] Casares-Marfil D, Strauss M, Bosch-Nicolau P, Presti MS, Molina I, Chevillard C, et al. A genome-wide association study identifies novel susceptibility loci in chronic Chagas cardiomyopathy. Clinical Infectious Diseases. 2021;**73**(4):672-679

[29] Clipman SJ, Henderson-Frost J, Fu KY, Bern C, Flores J, Gilman RH. Genetic association study of NLRP1, CARD, and CASP1 inflammasome genes with chronic Chagas cardiomyopathy among *Trypanosoma cruzi* seropositive patients in Bolivia. PLoS One. 2018;**13**(2):e0192378

[30] Steindel M, Kramer Pacheco L, Scholl D, Soares M, de Moraes MH, Eger I, et al. Characterization of *Trypanosoma cruzi* isolated from humans, vectors, and animal reservoirs following an outbreak of acute human Chagas disease in Santa Catarina state, Brazil. Diagnostic Microbiology and Infectious Disease. 2008;**60**(1):25-32. Available from: https://pubmed.ncbi.nlm.nih.gov/17889480/

[31] Silva CV, Luquetti AO, Rassi A, Mortara RA. Involvement of Ssp-4-related carbohydrate epitopes in mammalian cell invasion by *Trypanosoma cruzi* amastigotes. Microbes and Infection. 2006;**8**(8):2120-2129

[32] Pizzi T, Prager R. Estabilización de la virulencia de una cepa de *Trypanosoma cruzi* por pasaje seriado en ratones de constitución genética uniforme: análises cuantitativo del curso de la infección. Biologicals. 1952;**16**(17):3-12

[33] Liddell FD. Evaluation of survival in challenge experiments. Microbiological Reviews. 1978;**42**(1):237-249

[34] Langeron M. Précis de microscopie: Technique, expérimentation, diagnostic. Paris: Masson éditeurs; 1949

[35] Lagrange PH, Mackaness GB. A stable form of delayed-type hypersensitivity. The Journal of Experimental Medicine. 1975;**141**(1):82-96

[36] Sambrook J, Russell DW. Purification of nucleic acids by extraction with phenol:Chloroform. Cold Spring Harbor Protocols. 2006;**2006**(1):pdb.prot4455. Available from: https://pubmed.ncbi.nlm.nih.gov/22485786/

[37] Piron M, Fisa R, Casamitjana N, López-Chejade P, Puig L, Vergés M, et al. Development of a real-time PCR assay for *Trypanosoma cruzi* detection in blood samples. Acta Tropica. 2007;**103**(3):195-200

[38] Giulietti A, Overbergh L, Valckx D, Decallonne B, Bouillon R, Mathieu C. An overview of real-time quantitative PCR: Applications to quantify cytokine gene expression. Methods. 2001;**25**(4):386-401

[39] Barreto-de-Albuquerque J, Silva-dos-Santos D, Pérez AR, Berbert LR, de Santana-van-Vliet E, Farias-de-Oliveira DA, et al. *Trypanosoma cruzi* infection through the oral route promotes a severe infection in mice: New disease form from an old infection? PLoS Neglected Tropical Diseases. 2015;**9**(6):e0003849

[40] de Noya BA, González ON. An ecological overview on the factors that drives to *Trypanosoma cruzi* oral transmission. Acta Tropica. 2015;**151**(1):94-102

[41] Benchimol Barbosa PR. The oral transmission of Chagas' disease: An acute form of infection responsible for regional outbreaks. International Journal of Cardiology. 2006;**112**(1):132-133

[42] JCP D. Notes about of *Trypanosoma cruzi* and yours bio-ecology characteristics with agents of the transmission by meals. Revista da Sociedade Brasileira de Medicina Tropical. 2022;**39**(4):370-375

[43] Franco-Paredes C, Villamil-Gómez WE, Schultz J, Henao-Martínez AF, Parra-Henao G, Rassi A, et al. A deadly feast: Elucidating the burden of orally acquired acute Chagas disease in Latin America – Public health and travel medicine importance. Travel Medicine and Infectious Disease. 2020;**1**(36):101565

[44] Barreto de Albuquerque J, Silva dos Santos D, Stein JV, de Meis J. Oral versus Intragastric inoculation: Similar pathways of *Trypanosoma cruzi* experimental infection? From target

tissues, parasite evasion, and immune response. Frontiers in Immunology. 2018;**9**:30100907. Available from: https://pubmed.ncbi.nlm.nih.gov/30100907/

[45] Camandaroba ELP, Pinheiro Lima CM, Andrade SG. Oral transmission of Chagas disease: Importance of *Trypanosoma cruzi* biodeme in the intragastric experimental infection. Revista do Instituto de Medicina Tropical de Sao Paulo. 2022;**44**(2):97-103

[46] Dias GBM, Gruendling AP, Araújo SM, Gomes ML, MJO T. Evolution of infection in mice inoculated by the oral route with different developmental forms of *Trypanosoma cruzi* I and II. Experimental Parasitology. 2013;**135**(3):511-517

[47] Marsden PD. *Trypanosoma cruzi* infections in CFI mice. II. Infections induced by different routes. Annals of Tropical Medicine and Parasitology. 1967;**61**(1):62-67

[48] Collins MH, Craft JM, Bustamante JM, Tarleton RL. Oral exposure to *Trypanosoma cruzi* elicits a systemic $CD8^+$ T cell response and protection against heterotopic challenge. Infection and Immunity. 2011;**79**(8):3397-3406. DOI: 10.1128/IAI.01080-10. [Epub May 31, 2011]

[49] Cunha-Neto E, Chevillard C. Chagas diseasecardiomyopathy:Immunopathology and genetics. In: Mediators of Inflammation. 2014. p. 2014

[50] Chevillard C, Nunes JPS, Frade AF, Almeida RR, Pandey RP, Nascimento MS, et al. Disease tolerance and pathogen resistance genes may underlie *Trypanosoma cruzi* persistence and differential progression to Chagas disease cardiomyopathy. Frontiers in immunology. 2018;**9**:2791

[51] Silva GK, Cunha LD, Horta CV, Silva AL, Gutierrez FR, Silva JS, et al. A parent-of-origin effect determines the susceptibility of a non-informative F1 population to *Trypanosoma cruzi* infection in vivo. PLoS One. 2013;**8**(2):e56347. DOI: 10.1371/journal.pone.0056347. [Epub Feb 11, 2013]

[52] Hardoim D. Imunopatologia da infecção por *Trypanosoma cruzi* em camundongos CBA e C57BL/10 infectados pela vias intragástrica e intraperitoneal. 2014

[53] Ferreira BL, Ferreira ÉR, de Brito MV, Salu BR, MLV O, Mortara RA, et al. BALB/c and C57BL/6 mice cytokine responses to *Trypanosoma cruzi* infection are independent of parasite strain infectivity. Frontiers in Microbiology. 2018;**9**:1-12

[54] Bradley DJ. Genetic control of natural resistance to *Leishmania donovani*. Nature. 1974;**250**(5464):353

[55] Trammell RA, Liberati TA, Toth LA. Host genetic background and the innate inflammatory response of lung to influenza virus. Microbes and infection. 2012;**14**(1):50-58. Available from: https://pubmed.ncbi.nlm.nih.gov/21920449/

[56] von Köckritz-Blickwede M, Rohde M, Oehmcke S, Miller LS, CheungAL,HerwaldH,etal.Immunological mechanisms underlying the genetic predisposition to severe *Staphylococcus aureus* infection in the mouse model. The American Journal of Pathology. 2022;**173**(6):1657-1668. Available from: https://pubmed.ncbi.nlm.nih.gov/18974303/

[57] Malo D, Vogan K, Vidal S, Hu J, Cellier M, Schurr E, et al. Haplotype mapping and sequence analysis of the mouse Nramp gene predict susceptibility

to infection with intracellular parasites. Genomics. 1994;**23**(1):51-61

[58] Hedges JF, Kimmel E, Snyder DT, Jerome M, Jutila MA. Solute carrier 11A1 is expressed by innate lymphocytes and augments their activation. Journal of Immunology. 2013;**190**(8):4263-4273. Available from: https://pubmed.ncbi.nlm.nih.gov/23509347/

[59] de Góes Costa E, Dos Santos SO, Sojo-Milano M, Amador EC, Tatto E, Souza DS, et al. Acute Chagas disease in the Brazilian Amazon: Epidemiological and clinical features. International Journal of Cardiology. 2017;**235**:176-178. DOI: 10.1016/j.ijcard.2017.02.101. [Epub Feb 22, 2017]

[60] Casares-Marfil D, Kerick M, Andrés-León E, Bosch-Nicolau P, Molina I, Martin J, et al. GWAS loci associated with Chagas cardiomyopathy influences DNA methylation levels. PLoS Neglected Tropical Diseases. 2021;**15**(10)

[61] Cardoso JEZB. Hematological changes in mice experimentally infected with *Trypanosoma cruzi*. Memórias do Instituto Oswaldo Cruz. 1980;**75**:97-104

[62] Andrade SG, Rassi A, Magalhaes JB, F-FF, Luquetti A.O. Specific chemoterapy of Chagas disease: A comparison between the response in patients and experimental animals inoculated with the same strain. Transactions of the Royal Society of Tropical Medicine and Hygiene. 1992;**86**:624-626

[63] Malvezi AD, Cecchini R, de Souza F, Tadokoro CE, Rizzo LV, Pinge-Filho P. Involvement of nitric oxide (NO) and TNF-α in the oxidative stress associated with anemia in experimental *Trypanosoma cruzi* infection. FEMS Immunology and Medical Microbiology. 2004;**41**(1):69-77

[64] Miller LH, Good MF, Milon G, Miller LH, MFMG G. Malaria pathogenesis. Science. 1994;**264**(5167): 1878-1883

[65] Thomsen AR, Pisa P, Bro-Jorgensen K, KR. Mechanisms of lymphocytic choriomeningitis virusinduced hemopoietic dysfunction. Journal of Virology. 1986;**59**:428-433

[66] Rakusan TA. Inhibition of colony formation by human cytomegovirus in vitro. The Journal of Infectious Diseases. 1989;**159**:127-130

[67] Kaloutsi V, Kohlmeyer V, Maschet H, Nafe R, C, H., Amor A. GA. Comparison of bone marrow and hematological findings in patients with human immunodeficiency virus infection and those with myelodisplastic syndromes and infectious diseases. American Journal of Clinical Pathology. 1994;**101**:123-129

[68] Watier H, Verwaerde C, Landau I, Werner E, FJ, Capron A. AC. T cell-dependent immunity and thrombocytopenia in rats infected with *plasmodium chabaudi*. Infection and Immunity. 1992;**60**:136-142

[69] Davis CE, Robbins RS, Weller RDBAI. Thrombocytopenia in experimental trypanosomiasis. The Journal of Clinical Investigation. 1974;**53**:1359-1367

[70] van Putten LM. The life span of red cells in the rat and the mouse as determined by labeling with DFP32 in vivo. Blood. 1958;**13**(8):789-794. Available from: https://ashpublications.org/blood/article-pdf/13/8/789/553486/789.pdf

[71] Binder D, van den Broek MF, Kägi D, Bluethmann H, Fehr J, Hengartner H, et al. Aplastic anemia rescued by exhaustion of cytokine-secreting CD8+

T cells in persistent infection with lymphocytic choriomeningitis virus. Journal of Experimental Medicine. 1998;**187**(11):1903-1920. Available from: https://pubmed.ncbi.nlm.nih.gov/9607930/

[72] Ben D, MMM C. Recombinant tumor necrosis factor enhances the proliferative responsiveness of murine peripheral macrophages to macrophage-Colony stimulating factor but inhibits their proliferative responsiveness to granulocyte-macrophage-Colony stimulating factor. Blood. 1990;**75**:1627-1632

[73] Moldawer LL, Marano MA, Wei H, Fong Y, Silen ML, Kuo G, et al. Cachectin/tumor necrosis factor-α alters red blood cell kinetics and induces anemia in vivo. The FASEB Journal. 1989;**3**(5):1637-1643. Available from: https://pubmed.ncbi.nlm.nih.gov/2784116/

[74] Ulich TR, Shin SS, Castillo J d. Haematologic effects of TNF. Research in Immunology. 1993;**144**:347-354. Available from: https://pubmed.ncbi.nlm.nih.gov/8278657/

[75] Young HA, Klinman DM, Reynolds DA, Grzegorzewski KJ, Nii A, Ward JM, et al. Bone marrow and thymus expression of interferon-gamma results in severe B-cell lineage reduction, T-cell lineage alterations, and hematopoietic progenitor deficiencies. Blood. 1997;**89**(2):583-595

[76] Villalba-Alemán E, Justinico DL, Sarandy MM, Novaes RD, Freitas MB, Gonçalves RV. Haematological alterations in non-human hosts infected with *Trypanosoma cruzi*: A systematic review. Parasitology. 2019;**146**(2):142-160

[77] Tribulatti MV, Mucci J, van Rooijen N, Leguizamón MS, Campetella O. The trans-sialidase from *Trypanosoma cruzi* induces thrombocytopenia during acute Chagas' disease by reducing the platelet sialic acid contents. Infection and Immunity. 2005;**73**(1):201-207. Available from: https://pubmed.ncbi.nlm.nih.gov/15618155/

[78] Henderson SE, Pfeiffer SC, Novak J, Peace TA. Large granular lymphocytosis in a cynomolgus macaque (*Macaca fascicularis*) with a subclinical *Trypanosoma cruzi* infection. Veterinary Clinical Pathology. 2020;**49**:1-7

[79] Bonecini-Almeida M, Galvão-Castro B, Pessoa HR, Pirmez C, Laranja F. Experimental Chagas's disease in rhesus monkeys. I. Clinical, parasitological, hematological and anatomo-pathological studies in the acute and indeterminate phase of the disease. Memórias do Instituto Oswaldo Cruz. 1990;**85**:163-171

[80] Marcos P, Guedes M, Vanja, Veloso M, Wilson T, Mineo P, et al. Hematological alterations during experimental canine infection by *Trypanosoma cruzi* Alterações hematológicas durante a infecção canina experimental por *Trypanosoma cruzi*. Revista Brasileira de Parasitologia Veterinária. 2020;**21**(2):151-156. Available from: www.cbpv.com.br/rbpv

[81] Barr SC, Gossett KA, Klei TR. Clinical, clinicopathologic, and parasitologic observations of trypanosomiasis in dogs infected with north American *Trypanosoma cruzi* isolates. American Journal of Veterinary Research. 1991;**52**(6):954-960

[82] Marcondes MCG, Borelli P, Yoshida N, Russo M. Acute *Trypanosoma cruzi* infection is associated with anemia, thrombocytopenia, leukopenia, and

bone marrow hypoplasia: Reversal by nifurtimox treatment. Microbes and Infection. 2000;**2**(4):347-352

[83] Sathler-Avelar R, Vitelli-Avelar DM, Elói-Santos SM, Gontijo ED, Teixeira-Carvalho A, Martins-Filho OA. Blood leukocytes from benznidazole-treated indeterminate chagas disease patients display an overall type-1-modulated cytokine profile upon short-term in vitro stimulation with *Trypanosoma cruzi* antigens. BMC Infectious Diseases. 2012;**12**:123. Available from: https://pubmed.ncbi.nlm.nih.gov/22625224/

[84] Guo S, Cobb D, Smeltz RB. T-bet inhibits the in vivo differentiation of parasite-specific CD4+ Th17 cells in a T cell-intrinsic manner. Journal of Immunology. 2009;**182**(10):6179-6186. Available from: https://pubmed.ncbi.nlm.nih.gov/19414771/

[85] Dutra WO, Gollob KJ, Pinto-Dias JC, Gazzinelli G, Correa-Oliveira R, Coffman RL, et al. Cytokine mRNA profile of peripheral blood mononuclear cells isolated from individuals with *Trypanosoma cruzi* chronic infection. Scandinavian Journal of Immunology. 1997;**45**(1):74-80. Available from: https://pubmed.ncbi.nlm.nih.gov/9010503/

[86] Guedes PMDM, Gutierrez FRS, Maia FL, Milanezi CM, Silva GK, Pavanelli WR, et al. IL-17 produced during *Trypanosoma cruzi* infection plays a central role in regulating parasite-induced myocarditis. PLoS Neglected Tropical Diseases. 2010;**4**(2):e604. Available from: https://pubmed.ncbi.nlm.nih.gov/20169058/

[87] Martin Rick Tarleton D, Martin D, Tarleton R, Tarleton RL, Heiges M, Brayer T, et al. Generation, specificity, and function of CD8 þ T cells in *Trypanosoma cruzi* infection. Immunological Reviews. 2004;**201**:304-317

[88] Mateus J, Pérez-Antón E, Lasso P, Egui A, Roa N, Carrilero B, et al. Antiparasitic treatment induces an improved CD8 + T cell response in chronic Chagasic patients. Journal of Immunology. 2017;**198**(8):3170-3180. Available from: https://pubmed.ncbi.nlm.nih.gov/28258194/

[89] Albareda MC, Laucella SA, Alvarez MG, Armenti AH, Bertochi G, Tarleton RL, et al. *Trypanosoma cruzi* modulates the profile of memory CD8+ T cells in chronic Chagas' disease patients. International Immunology. 2006;**18**(3):465-471

[90] Cardillo F, de Pinho RT, Antas PRZ, Mengel J. Immunity and immune modulation in *Trypanosoma cruzi* infection. Pathogens and Disease. 2015;**73**:ftv082. Available from: https://pubmed.ncbi.nlm.nih.gov/26438729/

[91] Sathler-Avelar R, Vitelli-Avelar DM, Mattoso-Barbosa AM, Perdigão-de-Oliveira M, Costa RP, Elói-Santos SM, et al. Phenotypic features of circulating leukocytes from non-human primates naturally infected with *Trypanosoma cruzi* resemble the major immunological findings observed in human Chagas disease. PLoS Neglected Tropical Diseases. 2016;**10**(1):e0004302. Available from: https://pubmed.ncbi.nlm.nih.gov/26808481/

[92] de Meis J, Morrot A, Farias-de-Oliveira DA, Villa-Verde DMS, Savino W. Differential regional immune response in Chagas disease. PLoS Neglected Tropical Diseases. 2009;**3**(7):e417. Available from: https://pubmed.ncbi.nlm.nih.gov/19582140/

[93] Morrot A, Barreto De Albuquerque J, Berbert LR, de Carvalho Pinto CE,

de Meis J, Savino W. Dynamics of lymphocyte populations during *Trypanosoma cruzi* infection: From Thymocyte depletion to differential cell expansion/contraction in peripheral lymphoid organs. Journal of Tropical Medicine. 2012;**2012**:747185. Available from: https://pubmed.ncbi.nlm.nih.gov/22505943/

[94] Padilla AM, Bustamante JM, Tarleton RL. CD8+ T cells in *Trypanosoma cruzi* infection. Current Opinion in Immunology. 2009;**21**(4):385-390. Available from: https://pubmed.ncbi.nlm.nih.gov/19646853/

[95] Dhiman M, Garg NJ. P47phox−/− mice are compromised in expansion and activation of CD8+ T cells and susceptible to *Trypanosoma cruzi* infection. PLoS Pathogens. 2014;**10**(12):e1004516. Available from: https://pubmed.ncbi.nlm.nih.gov/25474113/

[96] Lieke T, Graefe SEB, Klauenberg U, Fleischer B, Jacobs T. NK cells contribute to the control of *Trypanosoma cruzi* infection by killing free parasites by perforin-independent mechanisms. Infection and Immunity. 2004;**72**(12):6817-6825. Available from: https://pubmed.ncbi.nlm.nih.gov/15557602/

[97] Tarleton RL. CD8+ T cells in *Trypanosoma cruzi* infection. Seminars in Immunopathology. 2015;**37, 37**:233-238

[98] Caselna TTT, Cruvinel WM, Mesquita Junior D, Pereira AJA, AWS d S, LEC A, et al. da imunologia aos imunobiológicos. Sinopse de Reumatologia. 2008;**2**:35-57

[99] Pérez AR, Roggero E, Nicora A, Palazzi J, Besedovsky HO, del Rey A, et al. Thymus atrophy during *Trypanosoma cruzi* infection is caused by an immuno-endocrine imbalance. Brain, Behavior, and Immunity. 2007;**21**(7):890-900. Available from: https://pubmed.ncbi.nlm.nih.gov/17412557/

[100] Sardinha LR, Mosca T, Elias RM, Do Nascimento RS, Gonçalves LA, Bucci DZ, et al. The liver plays a major role in clearance and destruction of blood Trypomastigotes in *Trypanosoma cruzi* chronically infected mice. Correa-Oliveira R, editor. PLoS Neglected Tropical Diseases. 2010;4(1):e578. Available from: https://dx.plos.org/10.1371/journal.pntd.0000578

[101] Jenne CN, Kubes P. Immune surveillance by the liver. Nature Immunology. 2013;**14**(10):996-1006

[102] Kubes P, Jenne C. Immune responses in the liver. Annual Review of Immunology. 2018;**36**(1):247-277. Available from: https://pubmed.ncbi.nlm.nih.gov/29328785/

[103] Hoft DF, Eickhoff CS, Giddings OK, JRC V, Rodrigues MM. Trans-Sialidase recombinant protein mixed with CpG motif-containing Oligodeoxynucleotide induces protective mucosal and systemic *Trypanosoma cruzi* immunity involving CD8 + CTL and B cell-mediated cross-priming. The Journal of Immunology. 2007;**179**(10):6889-6900. Available from: https://pubmed.ncbi.nlm.nih.gov/17982080/

[104] Arantes JM, Francisco AF, de Abreu Vieira PM, Silva M, Araújo MSS, de Carvalho AT, et al. *Trypanosoma cruzi*: Desferrioxamine decreases mortality and parasitemia in infected mice through a trypanostatic effect. Experimental Parasitology. 2011;**128**(4):401-408. Available from: https://pubmed.ncbi.nlm.nih.gov/21620835/

[105] Cardillo F, Postol E, Nihei J, Aroeira LS, Nomizo A, Mengel J. B cells

modulate T cells so as to favour T helper type 1 and CD8 + T-cell responses in the acute phase of *Trypanosoma cruzi* infection. Immunology. 2007;**122**(4):584-595. Available from: https://pubmed.ncbi.nlm.nih.gov/17635611/

[106] Dominguez MR, Ersching J, Lemos R, Machado A, Bruna-Romero O, Rodrigues MM, et al. Re-circulation of lymphocytes mediated by sphingosine-1-phosphate receptor-1 contributes to resistance against experimental infection with the protozoan parasite *Trypanosoma cruzi*. Vaccine. 2012;**30**(18):2882-2891

[107] Miyazaki Y, Hamano S, Wang S, Shimanoe Y, Iwakura Y, Yoshida H. IL-17 is necessary for host protection against acute-phase *Trypanosoma cruzi* infection. The Journal of Immunology. 2010;**185**(2):1150-1157. Available from: https://pubmed.ncbi.nlm.nih.gov/20562260/

[108] Canavaci AMC, Sorgi CA, Martins VP, Morais FR, de Sousa ÉVG, Trindade BC, et al. The acute phase of *Trypanosoma cruzi* infection is attenuated in 5-lipoxygenase-deficient mice. Mediators of Inflammation. 2014;**2014**:893634. Available from: https://pubmed.ncbi.nlm.nih.gov/25165415/

[109] Esper L, Utsch L, Soriani FM, Brant F, Esteves Arantes RM, Campos CF, et al. Regulatory effects of IL-18 on cytokine profiles and development of myocarditis during *Trypanosoma cruzi* infection. Microbes and Infection. 2014;**16**(6):481-490. Available from: https://pubmed.ncbi.nlm.nih.gov/24704475/

[110] Sanmarco LM, Visconti LM, Eberhardt N, Ramello MC, Ponce NE, Spitale NB, et al. IL-6 improves the nitric oxide-induced cytotoxic CD8+ T cell dysfunction in human Chagas disease. Frontiers in Immunology. 2022;**7**:626. Available from: https://pubmed.ncbi.nlm.nih.gov/28066435/

[111] Hoft DF, Farrar PL, Kratz-Owens K, Shaffer D. Gastric invasion by *Trypanosoma cruzi* and induction of protective mucosal immune responses. Infection and Immunity. 1996;**64**(9):3800-3810

[112] Silva-dos-Santos D, Barreto-de-Albuquerque J, Guerra B, Moreira OC, Berbert LR, Ramos MT, et al. Unraveling Chagas disease transmission through the oral route: Gateways to *Trypanosoma cruzi* infection and target tissues. PLoS Neglected Tropical Diseases. 2017;**11**(4):e0005507. Available from: https://pubmed.ncbi.nlm.nih.gov/28379959/

[113] de Meis J, Barreto de Albuquerque J, Silva Dos Santos D, Farias-de-Oliveira DA, Berbert LR, Cotta-de-Almeida V, et al. *Trypanosoma cruzi* entrance through systemic or mucosal infection sites differentially modulates regional immune response following acute infection in mice. Frontiers in Immunology. 2013;**4**(JUL):216. Available from: http://www.ncbi.nlm.nih.gov/pubmed/23898334

[114] Andrade LO, Machado CRS, Chiari E, Pena SDJ, Macedo AM. *Trypanosoma cruzi*: Role of host genetic background in the differential tissue distribution of parasite clonal populations. Experimental Parasitology. 2002;**100**(4):269-275

[115] Rassi A, Rassi A, Marin-Neto JA. Chagas disease. The Lancet. 2010;**375**:1388-1402. Available from: http://www.thelancet.com/article/S014067361060061X/fulltext

[116] Castro-Sesquen YE, Gilman RH, Paico H, Yauri V, Angulo N, Ccopa F,

et al. Cell death and serum markers of collagen metabolism during cardiac remodeling in *Cavia porcellus* experimentally infected with *Trypanosoma cruzi*. PLoS Neglected Tropical Diseases. 2013;**7**(2):e1996. Available from: https://pubmed.ncbi.nlm.nih.gov/23409197/

[117] Opie LH, Commerford PJ, Gersh BJ, Pfeffer MA. Controversies in ventricular remodelling. Lancet. 2006;**367**(9507):356-367. Available from: https://pubmed.ncbi.nlm.nih.gov/16443044/

[118] Quijano-Hernández IA, Castro-Barcena A, Aparicio-Burgos E, Barbosa-Mireles MA, Cruz-Chan JV, Vázquez-Chagoyán JC, et al. Evaluation of clinical and immunopathological features of different infective doses of *Trypanosoma cruzi* in dogs during the acute phase. The Scientific World Journal. 2012;**2012**:635169. Available from: https://pubmed.ncbi.nlm.nih.gov/22547991/

Chapter 7

# Modulation of Host Cell Apoptosis by *Trypanosoma cruzi*: Repercussions in the Development of Chronic Chagasic Cardiomyopathy

*Fiordaliso Carolina Román-Carraro, Diego Maurizio Coria-Paredes, Arturo A. Wilkins-Rodríguez and Laila Gutiérrez-Kobeh*

## Abstract

*Trypanosoma cruzi* is an intracellular parasite, which causes Chagas disease, affecting millions of people throughout the world. *T. cruzi* can invade several cell types, among which macrophages and cardiomyocytes stand out. Chagas disease goes through two stages: acute and chronic. If it becomes chronic, its most severe form is the chagasic chronic cardiomyopathy, which accounts for most of the fatalities due to this disease. For parasites to persist for long enough in cells, they should evade several host immune responses, one of these being apoptosis. Apoptosis is a type of programmed cell death described as a well-ordered and silent collection of steps that inevitably lead cells to a noninflammatory death. Cells respond to infection by initiating their own death to combat the infection. As a result, several intracellular microorganisms have developed different strategies to overcome host cell apoptosis and persist inside cells. It has been shown that *T. cruzi* has the ability to inhibit host cells apoptosis and can also induce apoptosis of cells that combat the parasite such as cytotoxic T cells. The aim of this chapter is to present up-to-date information about the molecules and mechanisms engaged by *T. cruzi* to achieve this goal and how the modulation of apoptosis by *T. cruzi* reflects in the development of chronic chagasic cardiomyopathy.

**Keywords:** apoptosis, cardiomyocytes, chronic chagasic cardiomyopathy, macrophages, T lymphocytes, *Trypanosoma cruzi*



IntechOpen

## 1. Introduction

The long-neglected disease called American trypanosomiasis or Chagas disease (CD) was first described in 1909 by the Brazilian doctor Carlos Chagas and it currently affects millions of people throughout the world. Its causative agent is the protozoan parasite *Trypanosoma cruzi* (Kinetoplastidae: Trypanosomatidae) found in more than 150 species of domestic and wild mammals that act as reservoirs [1, 2]. There are several transmission routes to humans such as the inoculation of parasites present in the feces of a hematophagous insect vector of the Triatominae subfamily or consumption of contaminated food with these feces, blood transfusions, organ transplants, and congenital [3]. The infection has a self-limiting acute phase with evident or absent parasitemia and may go unnoticed in many infected individuals. Some patients succumb during the acute phase of the disease, while others develop an adaptive immune response that generally controls the infection. If the parasite cannot be completely eradicated, the infection can last a lifetime and, if left untreated, presents potentially life-threatening complications such as chronic chagasic cardiomyopathy (CCC), which can present itself in its acute form or after a latency period that can extend for decades [4]. The persistence of the parasite in the host for such long periods indicates that it must surpass the host's immune response mechanisms, of which apoptosis is among the most important. Interestingly, *T. cruzi* is capable of inducing or preventing apoptosis of host cells as needed [5]. In this work, we describe the basic aspects of Chagas disease and analyze the role of apoptosis in the infection by this protozoan parasite.

## 2. Epidemiology

CD is endemic in 21 countries in Latin America, from Mexico to the south of Argentina and Chile. Nevertheless, due to migrations and climate change, the disease has spread alarmingly to other parts of the world [6]. The World Health Organization (WHO) classifies this parasitic disease as a VBD (Vector-Borne Disease) that is among the unattended tropical diseases associated to extreme poverty in rural areas where the vectors are distributed, which favors their transmission route [7]. VBDs can be caused by bacteria, virus, and parasites, are usually transmitted by bloodsucker arthropods, represent 17% of all infectious diseases, and are prevalent in tropical and subtropical regions [8]. During the past three decades, the epidemiological overview of this disease has experienced important changes due to the implementation of vector control measures such as the use of pesticides and housing improvements [9]. In this respect, there has been a clear descent in the number of people infected by *T. cruzi*, going from 30 million in 1990 to 6–7 million currently infected. The incidence has also decreased from 700,000 estimated cases in 1990 to 30,000 cases per year in 2018. Furthermore, the mortality has gone down from 45,000 to 12,000 deaths in the same years [10, 11]. Despite all these efforts, CD continues to be an important health problem. Migration of asymptomatic people in chronic stage, who are unaware of their infection, has led to the spread of the disease to urban areas and nonendemic regions, increasing the frequency of cases in countries such as the United States, Japan, Australia, Spain, Italy, the United Kingdom, and other European countries where it is considered an emerging disease [6, 12]. In Latin America, Argentina (1,535,235), Brazil (1, 156, 821), and Mexico (876, 458) are the countries with the highest number of cases, followed by Bolivia with 607, 186 cases, making it the country with the highest prevalence, with an estimate between 6.8 and 18% of the population seropositive for *T. cruzi* [13]. Recent estimations suggest that there could be 300,000 infected people with *T. cruzi* in the United States [14]. A study performed in Los Angeles reported a seroprevalence of 5.2% among Latin American migrants who also presented cardiac abnormalities [15]. Outside of America, Spain is the most affected country. It is estimated that only in this country there could be more than 50,000 infected individuals, most of them South American immigrants [16].

## 3. *Trypanosoma cruzi* life cycle

*T. cruzi* goes through several developmental stages. Within the vector, it is possible to find epimastigotes and metacyclic trypomastigotes, while blood trypomastigotes and amastigotes are found in vertebrates [17]. The cycle starts when a triatomine acquires blood trypomastigotes by sucking blood from an infected mammal [2]. Inside the vector, in the medial posterior gut, trypomastigotes differentiate to epimastigotes and duplicate. Afterward, epimastigotes migrate to the rectum, where they differentiate to metacyclic trypomastigotes. During the bloodmeal, vectors defecate and expel metacyclic trypomastigotes in their droppings that infect the mammal through the site of the bite, fissures in the skin, or mucous membranes [3, 18]. Parasites invade macrophages and connective tissue cells close to the site of entry due to the action of surface glycoproteins involved in the anchoring/penetration process such as gp82, gp83, gp85, and Tc-85, as well as glycoinositolphospholipids (GIPLs) [19–23]. Once inside cells, parasites have the ability to escape from the phagolysosome because of the action of enzymes such as a trans-sialidase (TS) and a low pH-dependent pore-forming protein, which allow them to reach the cytosol, where metacyclic trypomastigotes differentiate to amastigotes, duplicate, and finally transform to blood trypomastigotes that lyse the cell [24, 25]. They have the ability to surpass host effector mechanisms due to the expression of surface molecules such as GP160 and calreticulin that allow them to evade the action of complement, and GPI-mucins, which act as an antigenic protective coat. This antigenic coat presents variations that partially explain the differences in virulence and immunomodulation among strains [24, 26]. Trypomastigotes disseminate via lymph and blood to other tissues being able to infect any nucleated cell, but with certain tropism to macrophages, muscle cells (cardiac, smooth, and skeletal), and nervous cells. The cycle is completed when another vector ingests infected blood [17].

## 4. Genetic diversity

Initially it was thought that *T. cruzi* was a highly clonal species that had experienced little genetic mixing during its evolution [27]. However, due to increasingly detailed studies of the structure of populations and nuclear and mitochondrial DNA of *T. cruzi*, it has been suggested that in addition to clonal propagation, there have been more recent and frequent hybridizations and genetic exchange than previously thought [28]. At present, there are six discrete typification units (DTU TcI-VI) accepted by international consensus [29] that include at least two hybrid lineages (TcV and TcVI) and an additional one mainly found in bats (TcBat) [30, 31], closely related to TcI. Among these DTUs, TcI is the most diverse and widely distributed lineage with the smallest genome, the least amount of aneuploidy, and probably related with some hybrid lineages [28]. The association of a particular *T. cruzi* strain with the diverse spectrum of the disease has not been completely established [32], although it has been possible to show some correlations. For example, Chagas disease megasyndrome is mainly found in South America where TcV and TcVI predominate. On the other hand, in North and Central America, cardiomyopathy is more common with Tc1 being strongly associated with human infection [33].

## 5. Chagas disease

In humans, Chagas disease progresses through two phases, acute and chronic, with the development of a symptomatic or an asymptomatic form [34]. The initial acute phase evolves within 1–2 weeks after the inoculation, lasts for 4–8 weeks, and is characterized for high levels of blood parasitemia. Affected individuals show moderate and unspecific symptoms such as fever, general discomfort, and hepatosplenomegaly. Sometimes it is possible to observe a cutaneous node (inoculation chagoma) or a unilateral bipalpebral edema (Romaña sign) that indicates the parasite inoculation site [34, 35]. The majority of acute infections are never detected. Only in less than 1% of the cases, encephalitis or myocarditis occurs that can be fatal mainly in children and the elderly [36]. The initial increase in parasitemia is contained by proinflammatory cytokines (IL-12, TNF-α, IFN-γ) and microbicidal substances synthesized by macrophages (reactive oxygen and nitrogen species) and NK cells (perforins). This initial innate immune response is followed by the development of an acquired immune response characterized by a polyclonal lymphocyte activation against the parasite mediated by T $CD4^+$, $CD8^+$, and B lymphocytes, which together reduce the parasite load, but do not completely eliminate *T. cruzi*, which still survives in the host tissues, thus initiating the chronic phase [37, 38]. Observations from research conducted before 1990 show that after being in the acute phase for 10–30 years, 30–40% of patients will turn to the symptomatic chronic phase and present digestive and/or cardiac compromise, while the rest will remain in an indeterminate phase for the rest of their lives [39–41]. Recent studies performed in children and teenagers from endemic areas in Mexico suggest that the time for the outcome of the CCC symptoms is shorter, months in some cases. Therefore, more research is required to clarify this aspect [42, 43].

### 5.1 Gastronitestinal form of Chagas disease

The gastrointestinal form of Chagas disease affects the whole digestive tract, with the esophagus and colon being the most altered. They present anatomic and motor disturbances as a result of chronic inflammatory lesions, focal myositis, fibrosis, and damage to intramural neurons [44], which in the esophagus could lead to dysphagia, odynophagia, epigastric or retrosternal pain, cough, and regurgitation. In advanced stages, the denervated esophagus is unable to transport the bolus, retaining it at the level of the cardia, which can cause weight loss, malnutrition, and repetitive aspiration pneumonitis [46]. On the other hand, the megacolon is characterized by prolonged constipation that could lead to fecaloma, abdominal distension, and intestinal obstruction. Despite treatment with laxatives, patients worsen and may suffer from volvulus due to intestine torsion [45, 47].

### 5.2 Chagasic chronic cardiomyopathy

The chronic chagasic cardiomyopathy is the most critical clinical manifestation of Chagas disease due to its high morbidity and mortality in endemic regions [48, 49]. It is characterized by a complex pathogenesis, and many aspects are still under investigation. The causes for the colossal cardiac damage experienced by CCC patients have not been thoroughly explained, and different theories have been exposed throughout the years. It was previously thought that the cardiac damage was only caused by the direct action of the parasite over cardiomyocytes; however, it is now known that there are other contributing factors such as inflammatory response, autoimmunity, microvascular abnormalities, and nervous damage [50]. The cardiac tissue damage is progressive and characterized by chronic inflammation, myocytolysis, and fibrosis [51]. A recent study revealed that during a *T. cruzi* infection, activated macrophages release the metalloproteinases MMP2 and MMP9 that activate TGF-β signaling for cardiac extracellular remodeling and thus fibroblast differentiation to myofibroblasts that is a cellular phenotype present during damage and possesses characteristics that make it suitable for healing functions [51].

The most critical heart lesions are located in the myocardium and can lead to heart failure, arrhythmias, and thromboembolism. The heart excite-conducting system is also affected, blocking completely or incompletely some of the branches of the bundle of His (mainly the right) and sometimes a complete blockade of the atrioventricular node [50, 52].

The number of parasites in the cardiac tissue of CCC patients is scarce. This, together with the finding of immunoglobulins with affinity to muscarinic receptors and β-1 adrenergic expressed in the cardiomyocyte surface and the appearance of cytotoxic T lymphocytes with reactivity toward myocardial fibers, suggested that the etiology of CCC was autoimmune [53–57]. Investigations performed during the last 30 years in animal models infected with *T. cruzi* and patients with Chagas disease have modified this theory. Nowadays it is known that the amount of *T. cruzi* antigens correlates with the intensity of the inflammatory infiltrate that acts against the parasites that reside in the tissue [58]. Such infiltrate is mainly composed of macrophages and $CD8^+$ and $CD4^+$ T lymphocytes (2:1 ratio) that show a Th1 cytokine profile (TNF-α, IFN-γ, IL-1, IL-2) [59–61]. At first, this Th1 response protects the host, but its exacerbation produces diffuse myocarditis that over time causes myocytolysis and reparative fibrosis with interstitial deposition of collagen fibers, whose progression is directly correlated with cardiac dilatation and deterioration of systolic function. The growth of the left ventricle is common, although it is also possible to observe it in the right ventricle and auricles [52, 62]. In advanced stages of the disease, it is possible to find a cardiac apical aneurism, pathognomonic of CCC [49]. Studies carried out in patients and postmortem analysis have demonstrated the presence of intracavitary thrombi accompanied by infarcts in several organs such as the lungs, kidneys, and brain [63–65].

At present, the factors that contribute to the progression of patients from the indeterminate phase to the determinate phase of Chagas disease have not been fully elucidated. As for other infectious diseases, the prognosis of CD depends on factors attributable to the host and the pathogen. Being an intracellular parasite, *T. cruzi* needs to modulate the defense mechanisms of the host cell in order to guarantee its survival. One of these mechanisms is apoptosis.

## 6. Apoptosis

The word apoptosis has its etymological origin in the Greek apó, which means "from" and ptosis, which means "falling off." The term encompasses a genetically regulated process of cell death through which a cell destroys itself [66] with the key participation of cysteine-dependent proteases called caspases that are specific for aspartic acid [67]. Caspases are functionally divided in initiator (caspases 8, 9, and 10) and executioner (caspases 3, 6, and 7) [68]. In metazoans, apoptosis is an essential step in a great variety of physiological events such as embryogenesis, tissue remodeling, and the elimination of damaged or non-functional cells [69].

The sequence of events that lead to apoptosis can be unchained by two main routes: the extrinsic and the intrinsic pathways [66]. The intrinsic pathway initiates with the binding of death ligands (TNF-α, Fas-L, among others), present in soluble form or in the surface of effector cells, to their respective death receptors localized in the membrane of target cells. This binding results in the recruitment of cytosolic factors into the cytoplasmic domains of the death receptor, forming the death-inducing signaling complex or DISC. Initiator caspases such as procaspase 8, 10, or both are recruited to the DISC where they are activated. Caspases 8 and 10 in turn activate the following caspases in the pathway [70].

On the other hand, the intrinsic pathway, also known as the mitochondrial pathway of apoptosis, can be induced by various factors such as environmental stress or absence of growth factors. In this pathway, the formation of pores in the outer mitochondrial membrane allows the release of cytochrome-c into the cytosol, as well as other molecules such as endonuclease-G and Bcl-2 proteins. The interaction between cytochrome c, procaspase 9, and protease activating factor 1 or APAF 1 stimulates the formation of a heptameric complex known as apoptosome, which recruits procaspase 9 molecules, activating them. Caspase 9 molecules proceed to activate the following procaspases that execute the pathway, inducing apoptosis [66, 70].

Cells that die by apoptosis undergo characteristic morphological and biochemical changes that include a reduction in size, the collapse of the cytoskeleton, the disassembly of the nuclear envelope, and the fragmentation and condensation of chromatin. There are changes in the cell membrane composition and structure. Phosphatidylserine (PS) is translocated to the outer face of the membrane and protrusions are formed that finally break into membrane-enclosed fragments called apoptotic bodies. The mitochondrial membrane also changes with the formation of pores in the outer sheath that provokes the loss of the membrane potential of this organelle. These traits are used to quantitatively assess apoptosis [71, 72]. In metazoans, apoptotic cells and cell fragments are rapidly recognized and phagocytosed by cells of the immune system such as macrophages, which efficiently recognize PS expressed on the membrane of apoptotic cells. This early removal of cellular debris prevents the inflammatory response [73].

## 7. Apoptosis-like death in *T. cruzi*

It may seem odd to think that single-celled organisms can undergo apoptosis themselves, but it is believed that this has benefits for the survival of the population and therefore of the species. Shortly after apoptosis was described in metazoans, Docampo et al., using transmission electron microscopy, observed cytoplasmic and nuclear features suggestive of apoptosis in epimastigotes of *T. cruzi* treated with β-lapachone, an o-naphthoquinone that inhibits the synthesis of DNA. Such alterations included plasma membrane blebbing, chromatin condensation, and mitochondrial membrane alterations [74]. In addition to Trypanosoma, apoptotic death has been described in other protozoan taxa such as *Plasmodium*, and *Leishmania* that show distinctive characteristics of apoptosis similar to those described in multicellular organisms; however, the mechanisms involved are not fully understood [75]. Since then, other research groups have reported the appearance of stress- and drug-induced apoptotic traits (DNA fragmentation, PS externalization, loss of mitochondrial membrane potential, and cytochrome-c release) in *T. cruzi* [76, 77] with phenotypic similarities between metazoan cell apoptosis and *T. cruzi* cell death, but also with important differences in the processes and molecules that participate in them. Although PS translocation is a remarkable apoptotic trait in mammalian cells, in *T. cruzi* seems to be a parasite strategy to counteract macrophage activation [78]. On the other hand, caspases, key participants in apoptosis, are not present in *T. cruzi*. Nevertheless, its genome contains the TcMCA3 and TcMCA5 genes that code for metacaspases, cysteine proteases structurally similar to caspases but, unlike the latter, they have specificity for basic amino acid residues and are dependent on millimolar concentrations of calcium [79, 80]. The TcMCA3 protein is expressed in the four main stages of the parasite (epimastigotes, metacyclic trypomastigotes, blood trypomastigotes, and amastigotes), while TcMCA 5 is only expressed in epimastigotes. Analysis performed by immunofluorescence has shown that the treatment of *T. cruzi* with human serum, to induce programmed cell death, provokes a change in the subcellular localization of both metacaspases translocating them to the nucleus [81]. It has been observed that the increase in the expression of TcMCA5 augments the sensitivity of epimastigotes to programmed cell death as compared with parasites that express it at physiological levels. For its part, TcMCA3 protects epimastigotes from natural cell death and seems to play an important role in the process of differentiation to infectious metacyclic trypomastigotes [81].

Another molecule that could play an important role in the regulation of apoptotic cell death in *T. cruzi* is the elongation factor-1 (EF-1). This molecule, usually found in the nucleus and cytoplasm of eukaryotic cells, is formed of two subunits (EF-1$\alpha$ and EF-$\beta\gamma\delta$), and plays an important role in protein synthesis and in processes such as mitosis and cell proliferation [82]. Using anti-TcEF-1$\alpha$ antibodies coupled with fluorescein isothiocyanate, it was possible to observe that TcEF-1$\alpha$ accumulates in the nucleus of *T. cruzi* epimastigotes cultured for more than 13 days, which also showed apoptotic traits [83]. Subsequent investigations revealed that changes in the expression levels of EF-1$\alpha$ modify the rate of apoptosis in a murine erythroleukemic cell line [84], which suggests that TcEF-1$\alpha$ could be a marker of apoptosis in *T. cruzi*. The similarities that have been found between mammalian apoptosis and the phenomenon observed in *T. cruzi* have led some researchers to call it "apoptosis-like cell death" [85]. Nevertheless, other authors have concluded that the type of death observed in *Trypanosoma* and other protozoan parasites does not have the characteristics of a regulated death, and it is more an incidental cell death or necrosis [86].

## 8. Apoptosis modulation by *T. cruzi*

### 8.1 Apoptosis induction

Being an obligate intracellular parasite, *T. cruzi* needs to modulate the immune response mechanisms of its host to complete its life cycle and guarantee its survival and propagation. One of these mechanisms is apoptosis that can be modulated by this parasite on several cell types such as lymphocytes, macrophages, and cardiomyocytes. Macrophages are one of the most important niches in the mammalian host for *T. cruzi* replication and they are crucial for the immune response against the parasite because, depending on the stimulus, can be classically or alternatively activated. Classically activated macrophages (M1) produce nitric oxide (NO) that has the ability to kill *T. cruzi*, whereas alternatively activated macrophages, belonging to the M2 spectrum, synthesize polyamines that participate in parasite proliferation [87, 88]. Thus, one of the most important mechanisms of protective immunity against *T. cruzi* is a Th1-type immune response mediated by $CD4^+$ and $CD8^+$ T lymphocytes that produce IFN-γ, which in turn activates macrophages toward a classical phenotype for the control of parasitemia [89]. In response to this, *T. cruzi* displays outstanding strategies to control the activation of macrophages and inhibit apoptosis such as a reduction in the production of toxic molecules, including NO and its derivatives [90, 91], and the escape from the parasitophorous vacuole [92]. One of the molecules involved in the interference with NO is phosphatidylserine (PS). Experimental evidence indicates that PS exposure is connected to the survival and reproduction of obligate intracellular parasites by inhibiting NO production from macrophages [93, 94]. This strategy has been demonstrated in the infection of murine macrophages activated with IFN-γ and LPS with *T. cruzi* where trypomastigotes expose PS in their membrane. PS expression promotes parasite engulfment by phagocytic cells, a significant decrease in the expression of NOS2, and an increase in the production of the anti-inflammatory cytokine TGF-β by the infected macrophages. This suggests that the exposure of PS by *T. cruzi* (an apoptotic trait) could be responsible for the induction of the anti-inflammatory response similar to that induced by apoptotic cells [78].

In addition to the exposure of PS in the surface of *T. cruzi*, other membrane components participate in the immune evasion strategies and are considered virulence factors. All stages of *T. cruzi* have in their plasma membrane glycoconjugates attached to the membrane via glycosylphosphatidylinositol (GPI) anchors such as GIPLs and GPI-anchored glycoproteins [95], transialidase, mucins, mucin-associated proteins, and gp63 metalloproteases. It has been shown that GIPLs, in the presence of IFN-γ, induce apoptosis in macrophages through the ceramide portion by a NO production-independent pathway [96]. Also, it has been revealed that the sialylation of GPI-mucins protects trypomastigotes from lytic antibodies and, most likely, from the action of complement [97]. The alpha galactosylceramide expressed by *T. cruzi* induces anergy in NK cells and an increase in IL-33 [5]. On the other hand, the trans-sialidase (TS) of *T. cruzi* is an enzyme that transfers sialic acid from glycoconjugates present in mammalian cells to the parasite surface favoring its pathogenesis due to the formation of adhesive and protective structures on its surface. Also, TS has been shown to induce apoptosis of cells of the immune system [96]. In the infections with *T. cruzi*, TS can be located on the surface of the parasite or it can be secreted away from the site of infection [98]. Experiments performed in mice where recombinant TS was administered showed that the enzyme is capable of inducing apoptosis of the thymus. Contrarily, mice treated with anti-TS neutralizing antibodies did not show abnormalities in the organ [99, 100]. Later on, these observations were corroborated with the TUNEL assay and found that apoptosis was activated by sialylation of the CD43 mucin, which is constitutively expressed on the surface of T lymphocytes and monocytes [97]. This effect was not observed in mice that were given lactitol, an inhibitor of the transferase activity of the enzyme [101].

The induction of apoptosis in macrophages infected with *T. cruzi* may represent a proliferative strategy. It has been shown that when macrophages are infected with *T. cruzi* and phagocytose apoptotic CD4⁺ T cells, there is an increase in parasite replication inside macrophages, which in turn undergo apoptosis releasing more infective forms of the parasite such as trypomastigotes and spheromastigotes [5]. As a response to infection, macrophages release TGF-β, IL-10, and PGE2, which together deactivate them, allowing the survival of the intracellular forms of the parasite, as has also been observed with *Leishmania* [102].

For decades, the immunological suppression that *T. cruzi* exerts on cells of the immune system such as $CD4^+$ and $CD8^+$ T lymphocytes has been studied in detail, both in murine models and in patients with Chagas disease. This suppression can be macrophage-dependent or independent. In the first case, the unfavorable environment for T $CD4^+$ cell proliferation during the acute phase of *T. cruzi* infection is due to the production of IFN-γ and NO by activated macrophages. In the second case, the suppression of $CD4^+$ is through the interaction of TCR and CD3. The elimination of these cells inhibits the production of IFN-γ, thus preventing classical macrophage activation and favoring the development of an M2 phenotype, which favors the persistence of the parasite [88].

Likewise, apoptosis triggers the release of anti-inflammatory cytokines such as IL-10 and TGF-β by phagocytes, allowing the parasite to survive and continue with the infection.

It has been observed that in patients with chagasic cardiomyopathy there is no proliferation of peripheral blood mononuclear cells due to the activation of induced-apoptosis (AICD) by *T. cruzi* antigens. This has been complemented by the observation of a higher percentage of apoptotic cells in the hearts of patients with cardiac damage as compared with asymptomatic patients. Experimental evidence shows that the induction of apoptosis in $CD4^+$ T cells occurs through the induction of Fas/FasL and the activation of the executioner caspases 3 and 8 [103]. The participation of Fas/Fas-L was verified by *in vivo* injection of anti-FasL antibodies, which blocked the induced apoptosis of $CD8^+$ T lymphocytes, improving the Th1 response against the parasite. Interestingly, the blockade of TNF-α and TRAIL with antibodies did not have the same effect [104]. The increase in Fas-L has also been observed in the serum of patients in a chronic phase with CCC symptoms indicating that apoptosis also takes place during this phase [105]. Patients with chagasic cardiomyopathy showed a reduction in the proliferative response of T lymphocytes, in addition to a high production of $CD4^+CD62L^-$ T cells and an increase in the intracellular production of TNF-α, as well as the expression of genes of the TNF/TNFR superfamilies and caspases [106].

### 8.2 Apoptosis inhibition

*T. cruzi* is also capable of inhibiting apoptosis in infected cells. In addition to macrophages and T cells, the parasite also infects cardiomyocytes. *In vitro* experiments performed on murine cardiomyocytes incubated with *T. cruzi* or cruzipain (a parasite cysteine protease) showed that both trypomastigotes and cruzipain promote cardiomyocyte survival when cultured in media containing minimal serum concentrations. This phenomenon was associated with increased phosphorylation of Akt kinase and increased expression of the antiapoptotic protein Bcl-2. Furthermore, cultures that were treated with cruzipain showed less caspase-3 activation despite serum deprivation, suggesting that this enzyme might be responsible for the antiapoptotic effect [107]. Additionally, Chuenkova and Pereira observed that Schwann cells infected with

*T. cruzi* trypomastigotes are capable of surviving the proapoptotic stimulus induced by TNF-α, TGF-β, and $H_2O_2$. They found that the neurotrophic factor derived from the parasite (PNDF, a GPI-anchored neuraminidase and TS) interacts with the Akt kinase, increasing the expression levels of this protein and inhibiting the expression of at least 3 genes encoding proapoptotic proteins such as Bax, caspase-9, and the FOXO transcription factor, which together promoted cell viability [108].

It has been recently shown that *T. cruzi* amastigotes induce apoptosis in cardiomyocytes due to overexpression of Bax and reduced expression of Bcl-2 linked to trypomastigotes and amastigotes, respectively. The transcription factor STAT3, but not STAT1, was found to be active in cardiomyocytes due to trypomastigote infection. In addition, the TLR7 gene was observed to be overexpressed in cardiomyocytes incubated with trypomastigotes, which indicates that the TLR receptor is involved in intracellular recognition [109].

### 8.3 Apoptosis modulation by *T. cruzi* in other tissues

In addition to the modulation of apoptosis by *T. cruzi* of its main host cells, similar effects have been observed in other cell types. It has been shown that during the infection with *T. cruzi*, the parasite is able to induce apoptosis in human chorionic villi [110]. Also, the parasite has been shown to have an antiproliferative activity on the malignant melanoma cell line B16-BL6 [111].

The coinfection of *T. cruzi* with HIV can cause meningoencephalitis since both pathogens infect astrocytes. Interestingly, infected astrocytes with *T. cruzi* or *T. cruzi* and HIV, but not with HIV alone, showed a decrease in cell death and IL-6 secretion, which has a protective effect against death. This suggests that *T. cruzi* can reduce the induction of cell death by HIV and even more affect the replication of the virus [112].

## 9. Conclusion

Numerous studies have been performed with the aim to understand the molecular basis of the survival of *T. cruzi* in its host. *T. cruzi* is an intracellular parasite that needs to surpass different defense mechanisms and a hostile environment to persist inside host cells. To achieve this goal, this protozoan has developed a wide array of strategies that target different mechanisms and molecules in the host. One of the mechanisms that *T. cruzi* modulates is apoptosis. It has been shown that the parasite has the ability to induce or inhibit apoptosis of different cells. The profound knowledge of these targets will allow the development of strategies capable of interfering with the development of the disease. It remains to be elucidated which signal transduction pathway or pathways are responsible for establishing this relationship.

## Acknowledgements

Dr. Fiordaliso Carolina Román Carraro is a recipient of a postdoctoral fellowship from Dirección General de Asuntos del Personal Académico, UNAM. M. in Sci. Diego Maurizio Coria Paredes is a Ph.D. student of Posgrado en Ciencias Biológicas, Facultad de Medicina, UNAM. This work was supported by grant number IN214522 from Papiit, DGAPA, UNAM and funding from División de Investigación, Facultad de Medicina, UNAM TO LGK.

## Conflict of interest

The authors declare no conflict of interest.

## Author details

Fiordaliso Carolina Román-Carraro[1†], Diego Maurizio Coria-Paredes[1,2†], Arturo A. Wilkins-Rodríguez[1] and Laila Gutiérrez-Kobeh[1*]

1 Research Unit UNAM-INC, Research Division, School of Medicine, National Autonomous University of Mexico, Mexico City, Mexico

2 Facultad de Medicina, Posgrado en Ciencias Biológicas, Unidad de Posgrado, UNAM, Ciudad Universitaria, Ciudad de México, Mexico

*Address all correspondence to: lgutierr@unam.mx

† These authors have contributed equally.

## References

[1] Lewinsohn R. Carlos Chagas and the discovery of Chagas's disease (American tripanosomiasis). Journal of the Royal Society of Medicine. 1981;**74**:451-455. DOI: 10.1177/014107688107400612

[2] Rassi A, Rassi A, Marcondes de Rezende J. American Trypanosomiasis (Chagas disease). Infectious Disease Clinics of North America. 2012;**26**: 275-291. DOI: 10.1016/j.idc.2012.03.002

[3] Rassi A, Rassi A, Marin-Neto JA. Chagas disease. Lancet. 2010;**375**:1388-1402. DOI: 10.1016/S0140-6736(10)60061-X

[4] Gascón J, Albajar P, Cañas E, Flores M, Prat JG, Herrera RN, et al. Diagnosis, management, and treatment of chronic Chagas' heart disease in areas where *Trypanosoma cruzi* infection is not endemic. Revista Española de Cardiología. 2007;**60**:285-293

[5] Decote-Ricardo D, Nunes MP, Morrot A, Freire-de-Lima CD. Implications of apoptosis for the phathogenesis of *Trypanosoma cruzi* infection. Frontiers in Immunology. 2017;**8**:518. DOI: 10.3389/fimmu.2017.00518

[6] Freitas-Lidani KC, Andrade FA, Bavia L, Damasceno FS, Beltrame MH, Messias-Reason IJ, et al. Chagas disease: From discovery to a worldwide health problem. Frontiers in Public Health. 2019;**49**:1-13. DOI: 10.3389/fpubh.2019.00166

[7] World Health Organization (WHO). 2019. Chagas disease (American trypanosomiasis). Available from: https://www.who.int/health-topics/chagas-disease#tab=tab_1

[8] Vieira CB, Praça YR, Bentes KLS, Santiago PB, Silva SMM, Silva GS, et al. Triatomines: Trypanosomatids, Bacteria, and viruses potential vectors? Frontiers in Cellular and Infection Microbiology. 2018;**8**:1-12. DOI: 10.3389/fcimb.2018.00405

[9] Ramsey JM, Schofield CJ. Control of Chagas disease vectors. Salud Pública de México. 2003;**45**:123-128. DOI: 10.1590/s0036-36342003000200010

[10] Rodríguez-Morales AJ, Von A, Franco-Paredes C. Achievements and challenges in controlling Chagas disease. Boletín Médico del Hospital Infantil de México. 2011;**68**:102-109

[11] Organización Panamericana de la Salud (OPS). 2020. Enfermedad de Chagas. Available from: https://www.paho.org/es/temas/enfermedad-chagas

[12] Klein N, Hurwitz I, Durvasula R. Globalization of Chagas disease: A growing concern in nonendemic countries. Epidemiology Research International. 2012;**7**:1-13. DOI: 10.1155/2012/136793

[13] World Health Organization. Chagas disease in Latin America: An epidemiological update based on 2010 estimates. Relevé Épidémiologique Hebdomadaire. 2015;**90**:33-43

[14] Traina MI, Hernandez S, Sanchez DR, Dufani J, Salih M, Abuhamidah AM, et al. Prevalence of Chagas disease in a U.S. population of Latin American immigrants with conduction abnormalities on electrocardiogram. PLoS Neglected Tropical Diseases. 2017;**11**:e0005244. DOI: 10.1371/journal.pntd.0005244

[15] Bern C, Montgomery SP. An estimate of the burden of Chagas disease in the United States. Clinical Infectious Diseases. 2009;**49**:e52-e54. DOI: 10.1086/605091

[16] Blasco-Hernández T, García-San Miguel L, Navaza B, Navarro M, Benito A. Knowledge and experiences of Chagas disease in Bolivian women living in Spain: A qualitative study. Global Health Action. 2016;**9**(1):30201. DOI: 10.3402/gha.v9.30201

[17] Onyekwelu KC. Life cycle of *Trypanosoma cruzi* in the invertebrate and the vertebrate hosts. In: Biology of *Trypanosoma Cruzi*. 1st ed. Rijeka: IntechOpen; 2019. DOI: 10.5772/intechopen.84639

[18] García ES, Genta FA, Azambuja P, Shaub GA. Interactions between intestinal compounds of triatomines and *Trypanosoma cruzi*. Trends in Parasitology. 2010;**26**:499-505. DOI: 10.1016/j.pt.2010.07.003

[19] Tardieux I, Nathanson MH, Andrews NW. Role in the host cell invasion of *Trypanosoma cruzi* induced cytosolic free $Ca^{2+}$ transients. Journal of Experimental Medicine. 1994;**179**:1017-1022. DOI: 10.1084/jem.179.3.1017

[20] Lima MF, Villalta F. Host-cell attachment by *Trypanosoma cruzi* identification of an adhesion molecule. Biochemical and Biophysical Research Communications. 1988;**155**:256-262. DOI: 10.1016/s0006-291x(88)81077-5

[21] Mattos EC, Tonelli RR, Colli W, Alves MJ. The Gp85 surface glycoproteins from Trypanosoma cruzi. Sub-cellular. Biochemistry. 2014;**74**:151-180. DOI: 10.1007/978-94-007-7305_9_7

[22] Colli W, Alves MJ. Relevant glycoconjugates on the surface of *Trypanosoma cruzi*. Memórias do Instituto Oswaldo Cruz. 1999;**94**:37-49. DOI: 10.1590/s0074-02761999000700004

[23] de Souza W, de Carvalho TM, Barrias ES. Review on *Trypanosoma cruzi*: Host cell interaction. International Journal of Cell Biology. 2010;**2010**:295394. DOI: 10.1155/2010/295394

[24] Cardoso MS, Reis-Cunha JL, Bartholomeu DC. Evasion of the immune response by *Trypanosoma cruzi* during acute infection. Frontiers in Immunology. 2016;**6**:659. DOI: 10.3389/fimmu.2015.00659

[25] Sibley LD, Andrews NW. Cell invasion by un-palatable parasites. Traffic. 2000;**1**:100-106. DOI: 10.1034/j.1600-0854.2000.010202.x

[26] Soares RP, Torrecilhas AC, Assis RR, Rocha MN, Moura E, Castro FA, et al. Intraspecies variation in *Trypanosoma cruzi* GPI-mucins: Biological activities and differential expression of α-galactosyl residues. American Journal of Tropical Medicine and Hygiene. 2012;**87**:87-96. DOI: 10.4269/ajtmh.2012.12-0015

[27] Tibayrenc M. Genetic subdivisions within *Trypanosoma cruzi* (discrete typing units) and their relevance for molecular epidemiology and experimental evolution. Kinetoplastid Biology and Disease. 2003;**2**:12. DOI: 10.1186/1475-9292-2-12

[28] Messenger LA, Miles MA. Evidence and importance of genetic exchange among field populations of *Trypanosoma cruzi*. Acta Tropica. 2015;**151**:150-155. DOI: 10.1016/j.actatropica.2015.05.007

[29] Zingales B, Miles MA, Campbell DA, Tibayrenc M, Macedo AM, Teixeira MM,

et al. The revised *Trypanosoma cruzi* subspecific nomenclature: Rationale, epidemiological relevance and research applications. Infection, Genetics and Evolution. 2012;**12**:240-253. DOI: 10.1016/j.meegid.2011.12.009

[30] Marcili A, Lima L, Cavazzana M, Junqueira AC, Veludo HH, Maia Da Silva F, et al. A new genotype of *Trypanosoma cruzi* associated with bats evidenced by phylogenetic analyses using SSU rDNA, cytochrome b and histone H2B genes and genotyping based on ITS1 rDNA. Parasitology. 2009;**136**:641-655. DOI: 10.1017/S0031182009005861

[31] Ramirez JD, Hernandez C, Montilla M, Zambrano P, Florez AC, Parra E, et al. First report of human *Trypanosoma cruzi* infection attributed to TcBat genotype. Zoonoses and Public Health. 2014;**61**:477-479. DOI: 10.1111/zph.12094

[32] Lewis MD, Francisco AF, Taylor MC, Jayawardhana S, Kelly JM. Host and parasite genetics shape a link between *Trypanosoma cruzi* infection dynamics and chronic cardiomyopathy. Cellular Microbiology. 2016;**18**:1429-1443. DOI: 10.1111/cmi.12584

[33] Gruendling AP, Massago M, Teston AP, Monteiro WM, Kaneshima EN, Araujo SM, et al. Impact of benznidazole on infection course in mice experimentally infected with *Trypanosoma cruzi* I, II, and IV. American Journal of Tropical Medicine and Hygiene. 2015;**92**:1178-1189. DOI: 10.4269/ajtmh.13-0690

[34] Bern C. Chagas' disease. New England Journal of Medicine. 2015;**373**:456-466. DOI: 10.1056/NEJMra1410150

[35] Malik LH, Singh GD, Amsterdam EA. The epidemiology, clinical manifestations, and management of Chagas heart disease. Clinical Cardiology. 2015;**38**:565-569. DOI: 10.1002/clc.22421

[36] Pérez-Molina JA, Molina I. Chagas disease. Lancet. 2018;**391**:82-94. DOI: 10.1016/S0140-6736(17)31612-4

[37] Acevedo GR, Girard MC, Gómez KA. The unsolved jigsaw puzzle of the immune response in Chagas disease. Frontiers in Immunology. 2018;**9**:1929. DOI: 10.3389/fimmu.2018.01929

[38] Reyes AC, Rosales JLE. *Trypanosoma cruzi* infection: Mechanisms of evasion of immune response. In: Biology of *Trypanosoma Cruzi*. 1st ed. Rijeka: IntechOpen; 2019. DOI: 10.5772/intechopen.84359

[39] Espinosa R, Carrasco HA, Belandria F, Fuenmayor AM, Molina C, González R, et al. Life expectancy analysis in patients with Chagas' disease: Prognosis after one decade (1973-1983). International Journal of Cardiology. 1985;**85**:45-56. DOI: 10.1016/0167-5273(85)90262-1

[40] Gascón J, Albajar P, Cañas E, Flores M, Gómez i Prat J, Herrera RN, Lafuente CA, Luciardi HL, Moncayo A, Molina L, Muñoz J, Puente S, Sanz G, Treviño B, Sergio-Salles X. Diagnosis, management and treatment of chronic Chagas' heart disease in areas where *Trypanosoma cruzi* is not endemic. Revista Española de Cardiología. 2007;**60**:285-293

[41] Rodriguez CJ, Borges-Pereira J. Chronic phase of Chagas disease: Why should it be treated? A comprehensive review. Memórias do Instituto Oswaldo Cruz. 2011;**106**:641-645. DOI: 10.1590/s0074-02762011000600001

[42] Salazar-Schettino PM, Cabrera-Bravo M, Vazquez-Antona C, Zenteno E,

de Alba-Alvarado M, Torres-Gutiérrez E, et al. Chagas disease in México: Report of 14 cases of Chagasic cardiomyopathy in children. The Tohoku Journal of Experimental Medicine. 2016;**240**:243-249. DOI: 10.1620/tjem.240.243

[43] Méndez-Dominguez N, Chi-Méndez C, Canto-Losa J, Peniche-Echazarreta A, Canto-Losa JP, Gómez-Carro S. Chagasic Cardiopathy in a child: Case report. Revista Chilena de Pediatría. 2017;**88**:647-651. DOI: 10.4067/S0370-41062017000500012

[44] Bilder CR, Goin JC. Gastrointestinal involvement in Chagas disease. Neurogastro Reviews LATAM. 2017;**1**:168-179

[45] Carrada-Bravo T. *Trypanosoma cruzi*: historia natural y diagnóstico de la enfermedad de Chagas. Revista Mexicana de Patología Clínica. 2004;**51**:205-219

[46] Matsuda NM, Miller SM, Evora PR. The chronic gastrointestinal manifestations of Chagas disease. Clinics (São Paulo, Brazil). 2009;**64**:1219-1224. DOI: 10.1590/S18075932200900 1200013

[47] Dias JC. The indeterminate form of human chronic Chagas'disease. A clinical epidemiological review. Revista da Sociedade Brasileira de Medicina Tropical. 1989;**22**:147-156. DOI: 10.1590/s0037-86821989000300007

[48] Hotez P, Bottazzi ME, Strub-Wourgaft N, Sosa-Estani S, Torrico F, Pajín L, et al. A new patient registry for Chagas disease. PLoS Neglected Tropical Diseases. 2020;**14**:e0008418. DOI: 10.1371/journal.pntd.0008418

[49] Pech-Aguilar AG, Haro-Álvarez AP, Rosado-Vallado ME. Updated review on the pathophysiology of Chagas cardiomyopathy. Revista Médica del Instituto Mexicano del Seguro Social. 2020;**58**:1-8. DOI: 10.24875/RMIMSS.M20000037

[50] Benck L, Kransdorf E, Patel J. Diagnosis and management of Chagas cardiomyopathy in the United States. Current Cardiology Reports. 2018;**20**:131. DOI: 10.1007/s11886-018-1077-5

[51] Choudhuri S, Garg NJ. *Trypanosoma cruzi* induces the parp1/ap-1 pathway for upregulation of metalloproteinases and transforming growth factor β in macrophages: Role in cardiac fibroblast differentiation and fibrosis in Chagas disease. MBio. 2020;**11**:e01853-e01820. DOI: 10.1128/mBio.01853-20

[52] Texeira AR, Nascimento RJ, Sturn NR. Evolution and pathology in Chagas disease-a review. Memórias do Instituto Oswaldo Cruz. 2006;**101**:463-491. DOI: 10.1590/s0074-02762006000500001

[53] Cossio PM, Diez C, Szarfman A. Chagasic cardiopathy. Demonstration of a serum gamma globulin factor which reacts with endocardium and vascular structures. Circulation. 1974;**49**:13-21. DOI: 10.1161/01.cir.49.1.13

[54] Higuchi ML, Lopes EA, Saldanha LB, Barretto AC, Stolf NA, Bellotti G, et al. Immunopathologic studies in myocardial biopsies of patients with Chagas disease and idiopathic cardiomyopathy. Revista do Instituto de Medicina Tropical de São Paulo. 1986;**28**:87-90. DOI: 10.1590/s0036-46651986000200004

[55] Borda EP, Cossio P, Veja MV, Arana R, Sterin-Borda L. A circulating IgG in Chagas disease which binds to β-adrenoreceptors of myocardium and modulates their activity. Clinical and Experimental Immunology. 1984;**57**:679-686

[56] Sterin-Borda L, Gorelik G, Borda ES. Chagasic IgG binding with cardiac

muscarinic cholinergic receptors modifies cholinergic-mediated cellular transmembrane signals. Clinical Immunology and Immunopathology. 1991;**61**:387-397. DOI: 10.1016/s0090-1229(05)80010-8

[57] Santos-Buch CA, Texeira AR. The immunology of experimental Chagas' disease. III. Rejection of allogeneic hearth cells in vitro. Journal of Experimental Medicine. 1974;**140**:38-53. DOI: 10.1084/jem.140.1.38

[58] Higuchi MDL, Reis MM, Aiello VD, Benvenuti LA, Gutierrez PS, Belloti G, et al. Association of an increase in CD8$^+$ T cells with the presence of *Trypanosoma cruzi* antigens in chronic, human, chagasic myocarditis. American Journal of Tropical Medicine and Hygiene. 1997;**56**:485-489. DOI: 10.4269/ajtmh.1997.56.485

[59] Higuchi MDL, Gutiérrez VDA. Immunohistochemical characterization of infiltrating cell in human chronic chagasic myocarditis: Comparison with myocardial rejection process. Virchows Archiv. A, Pathological Anatomy and Histopathology. 1993;**423**:157-160. DOI: 10.1007/BF01614765

[60] Morato MJF, Colley DG, dos Reis MA. Cytokines profiles during experimental Chagas' disease. Brazilian Journal of Medical and Biological Research. 1998;**31**:123-125. DOI: 10.1590/s0100-879x1998000100016

[61] Rocha-Rodrigues DB, Dos Reis MA, Romano A, de Lima SA, Antunes V, Tostes S, et al. In situ expression of regulatory cytokines by heart inflammatory cells in Chagas' disease patients with hearth failure. Clinical and Developmental Immunology. 2012;**2012**:361730. DOI: 10.1155/2012/361730

[62] Rossi MA. The pattern of myocardial fibrosis in chronic Chagas' heart disease. International Journal of Cardiology. 1991;**30**:335-340. DOI: 10.1016/0167-5273(91)90012-e

[63] Bezerra da Silva G, Hörbe Antunes V, Motta M, et al. Chagas disease-associated kidney injury – A review. Nefrología Latinoamericana. 2017;**22**:22-26

[64] Carod-Artal FJ. Stroke: A neglected complication of American trypanosomiasis (Chagas' disease). Transactions of the Royal Society of Tropical Medicine and Hygiene. 2007;**102**:1075-1080. DOI: 10.1016/j.trstmh.2007.06.007

[65] Samuel J, Oliveira M, Correa De Araujo RR, Navarro MA, Muccillo G. Cardiac thrombosis and thromboembolism in chronic Chagas' heart disease. The American Journal of Cardiology. 1983;**52**:147-151. DOI: 10.1016/0002-9149(83)90085-1

[66] Elmore S. Apoptosis: A review of programmed cell death. Toxicologic Pathology. 2007;**35**:495-516. DOI: 10.1080/01926230701320337

[67] Keller N, Grüter M, Zerbe O. Studies of the molecular mechanism of caspase-8 activation by solution NMR. Cell Death and Differentiation. 2010;**17**:710-718. DOI: 10.1038/cdd.2009.155

[68] Opdenbosch NV, Lamkanfi M. Caspases in cell death, inflammation, and disease. Immunity. 2019;**50**:1352-1364. DOI: 10.1016/j.immuni.2019.05.020

[69] Singh R, Letai A, Sarosiek K. Regulation of apoptosis in health and disease: The balancing act of BCL-2 family proteins. Nature Reviews Molecular Cell Biology. 2019;**20**:175-193. DOI: 10.1038/s41580-018-0089-8

[70] D'Arcy MS. Cell death. A review of the major forms of apoptosis, necrosis and autophagy. Cell Biology International. 2019;**43**:582-592. DOI: 10.1002/cbin.11137

[71] Saraste A, Pulkki K. Morphologic and biochemical hallmarks of apoptosis. Cardiovascular Research. 2000;**45**:528-537. DOI: 10.1016/s0008-6393(99)00384-3

[72] Galluzzi L, Vitale I, et al. Molecular mechanisms of cell death: Recommendations of the nomenclature committee on cell death. Cell Death and Differentiation. 2018;**25**:486-541. DOI: 10.1038/s41418-017-0012-4

[73] Henson PM, Bratton DL, Fadok VA. Apoptotic cell removal. Current Biology. 2001;**11**:R795-R805. DOI: 10.1016/S0960-9822(01)00474-2

[74] Docampo R, Lopes JN, Cruz FS, de Souza W. *Trypanosoma cruzi*: Ultrastructural and metabolic alterations of epimastigotes by β-lapachone. Experimental Parasitology. 1977;**42**:142-149. DOI: 10.1016/0014-4894(77)90071-6

[75] Kaczanowski S. Apoptosis: Its origin, history, maintenance and the medical implications for cancer and aging. Physical Biology. 2016;**13**:031001. DOI: 10.1088/1478-3975/13/3/031001

[76] Piacenza L, Peluffo G, Radi R. L-arginine-dependent suppression of apoptosis in *Trypanosoma cruzi*: Contribution of the nitric oxide and polyamine pathways. Proceedings of the National Academy of Sciences of the United States of America. 2001;**98**:7301-7306. DOI: 10.1073/pnas.121520398

[77] Zuma AA, Mendes IC, Reignault LC, Elias MC, de Souza W, Machado CR, et al. How *Trypanosoma cruzi* handles cell cycle arrest promoted by camptothecin, a topoisomerase I inhibitor. Molecular and Biochemical Parasitology. 2014;**193**:93-100. DOI: 10.1016/j.molbiopara.2014.02.001

[78] Damatta RA, Seabra SH, Deolindo P, Arnholdt ACV, Manhães L, Goldenberg S, et al. *Trypanosoma cruzi* exposes phosphatidylserine as an evasion mechanism. FEMS Microbiology Letters. 2006;**266**:29-33. DOI: 10.1111/j.1514-6968.2006.00495.x

[79] Kosec G, Alvarez VE, Agüero F, Sánchez D, Dolinar M, Turk B, et al. Metacaspases of *Trypanosoma cruzi*: Possible candidates for programmed cell death mediators. Molecular and Biochemical Parasitology. 2006;**145**:18-28. DOI: 10.1016/j.molbiopara.2005.09.001

[80] Uren AG, O'Rourke K, Aravind L, Pisabarro MT, Seshagiri S, Koonin EV, et al. Identification of paracaspases and metacaspases: Two ancient families of caspase-like proteins, one of which plays a key role in MALT-lymphoma. Molecular Cell. 2002;**9**:911-917. DOI: 10.1016/s1097-2765(00)00094-0

[81] Laverrière M, Cazzulo JJ, Alvarez VE. Antagonic activities of *Trypanosoma cruzi* metacaspases affect the balance between cell proliferation, death and differentiation. Cell Death and Differentation. 2012;**19**:1358-1369. DOI: 10.1038/cdd.2012.12

[82] Sasikumar AN, Perez WB, Kinzy TG. The many roles of the eukaryotic elongation factor 1 complex. Wiley Interdisciplinary Reviews: RNA. 2012;**3**:543-555. DOI: 10.1002/wrna.1118

[83] Billaut-Mulot O, Fernández-Gómez R, Loyens M, Ouaissi A.

*Trypanosoma cruzi* elongation factor 1α: Nuclear localization in parasites undergoing apoptosis. Gene. 1996;**174**:19-26. DOI: 10.1016/0378-1119(96)00254-5

[84] Kato MV. The mechanisms of death of an erythroleukemic cell line by p53: Involvement of the microtubule and mitochondria. Leukemia and Lymphoma. 1999;**33**:181-186. DOI: 10.3109/10428199909093740

[85] Menna-Barreto RFS. Cell death pathways in pathogenic trypanosomatids: Lessons of (over) kill. Cell Death & Disease. 2019;**10**:93. DOI: 10.1038/s41419-019-1370-2

[86] Proto WR, Coombs GH, Mottram JC. Cell death in parasitic protozoa: regulated or incidental? Nature Reviews Microbiology. 2013;**11**:58-66. DOI: 10.1038/nrmicro2929

[87] Mills CD, Kincaid K, Alt JM, Heilman MJ, Hill AM. M-1/M-2 macrophages and the Th1/Th2 paradigm. Journal of Immunology. 2000;**164**:6166-6173. DOI: 10.4049/jimmunol.164.12.6166

[88] Bastos KR, Alvarez JM, Marinho CR, Rizzo LV, Lima MR. Macrophages from IL-12p40-deficient mice have a bias toward the M2 activation profile. Journal of Leukocyte Biology. 2002;**71**:271-278

[89] Ghabdan-Zanluqui N, Fanini-Wowk P, Pinge-Filho P. Macrophage polarization in Chagas disease. Journal of Clinical and Cellular Immunology. 2015;**6**:2. DOI: 10.4172/2155-9899.1000317

[90] Vincendeau P, Daulouède S. Macrophage cytostatic efect on Trypanosoma musculi involves an L-arginine-dependent mechanism. Journal of Immunology. 1991;**146**:4338-4343

[91] Bogdan C. Nitric oxide synthase in innate and adaptive immunity: An update. Trends in Immunology. 2015;**36**:161-178. DOI: 10.1016/j.it.2015.01.003

[92] Nogueira N, Cohn Z. Trypanosoma cruzi: Mechanism of entry and intracellular fate in mammalian cells. Journal of Experimental Medicine. 1976;**143**:1402-1420. DOI: 10.1084/jem.143.6.1402

[93] Seabra SH, de Souza W, DaMatta RA. *Toxoplasma gondii* exposes phophatidylserine that induces a TGF-β autocrine effect orchestrating macrophages evasion. Biochemical and Biophysical Research Communications. 2004;**324**:744-752. DOI: 10.1016/j.bbrc.2004.09.114

[94] Wanderley JL, Moreira ME, Benjamin A, Bonomo AC, Barcinski MA. Mimicry of apoptotic cells by exposing phosphatidylserine participes in the establishment of amastigotes of *Leishmania (L) amazonensis* in mammalian hosts. Journal of Immunology. 2006;**176**:1834-1839. DOI: 10.4049/jimmunol.176.3.1834

[95] Figueiredo JM, Rodrigues DC, Silva RC, Koeller CM, Jiang JC, Jazwinski MS, et al. Molecular and functional characterization of the ceramide synthase from Trypanosoma cruzi. Molecular and Biochemical Parasitology. 2013;**182**:62-74. DOI: 10.1016/j.molbiopara.2011.12.006

[96] Booth L, Smith TK, Booth L, Smith TK. Lipid metabolism in *Trypanosoma cruzi*: A review. Molecular and Biochemical Parasitology. 2020;**240**:111324. DOI: 10.1016/j.molbiopara.2020.111324

[97] Mucci J, Risso MG, Leguizamón MS, Frasch ACC, Campetella O. The trans -sialidase from *Trypanosoma cruzi* triggers apoptosis by target cell sialylation. Cellular Microbiology. 2006;**8**:1086-1095. DOI: 10.1111/j.1462-5822.2006.00689.x

[98] Buschiazzo A, Amaya MF, Cremona ML, Frasch AC, Alzari PM. The crystal structure and mode of action of trans-sialidase, a key enzyme in *Trypanosoma cruzi* pathogenesis. Molecular Cell. 2002;**10**:757-768. DOI: 10.1016/s1097-2765(02)00680-9

[99] Leguizamón MS, Mocetti E, Garcia-Rivello H, Argibay PF, Campetella O. *Trans*-sialidase from *Trypanosoma cruzi* induces apoptosis in cells from the immune system *in vivo*. Journal of Infectious Diseases. 1999;**180**:1398-1402. DOI: 10.1086/315001

[100] Mucci J, Hidalgo A, Mocetti E, Argibay PF, Leguizamón MS, Campetella O. Thymocyte depletion in *Trypanosoma cruzi* infection is mediated by *trans*-sialidase induced apoptosis on nurse cells complex. Proceedings of the National Academy of Sciences of the United States of America. 2002;**99**:3896-3901. DOI: 10.1073/pnas.052496399

[101] Aoki M, Guiñazú NL, Pellegrini AV, Gotoh T, Masih DT, Gea S. Cruzipain, a major *Trypanosoma cruzi* antigen, promotes arginase-2 expression and survival of neonatal mouse cardiomyocytes. American Journal of Physiology. Cell Physiology. 2004;**286**:C206-C212. DOI: 10.1152/ajpcell.00282.2003

[102] Arcanjo AF, LaRocque-de-Freitas IF, Rocha JDB, Zamith D, Costa-da-Silva AC, Nunes MP, et al. The PGE2/IL-10 axis determines susceptibility of B-1 cell-derived phagocytes (B-1CDP) to *Leishmania major* infection. PLoS One. 2015;**10**:1-18. DOI: 10.1371/journal.pone.0124888

[103] Lopes MF, Nunes MP, Henriques-Pons A, Giese N, Morse HC III, Davidson WF, et al. Increased susceptibility of Fas ligand-deficient gld mice to *Trypanosoma cruzi* infection due to a Th2-biased host immune response. European Journal of Immunology. 1999;**29**:81-89. DOI: 10.1002/(SICI)1521-4141(199901)29:01<81::AID-IMMU81>3.0.CO;2-Y

[104] Guillermo LV, Silva EM, Ribeiro-Gomes FL, De Meis J, Pereira WF, Yagita H, et al. The Fas death pathway controls coordinated expansions of type 1 CD8 and type 2 CD4 T cells in Trypanosoma cruzi infection. Journal of Leukocyte Biology. 2007;**81**:942-951. DOI: 10.1189/jlb.1006643

[105] Rodrigues V Jr, Agrelli GS, Leon SC, Silva Texeira DN, Tostes S Jr, Rocha-Rodrigues DB. Fas/Fas-L expression, apoptosis and low proliferative response are associated with hearth failure in patients with chronic Chagas' disease. Microbes and Infection. 2008;**10**:29-37. DOI: 10.1016/j.micinf.2007.09.015

[106] Chaves AT, Assis J, De Gomes S, Fiuza JA, Carvalho AT, Ferreira KS, et al. Immunoregulatory mechanisms in Chagas disease: Modulation of apoptosis in T-cell mediated immune responses. BMC Infectious Diseases. 2016;**16**:1-11. DOI: 10.1186/s12879-016-1523-1

[107] Chuenkova MV, Pereira PM. *Trypanosoma cruzi* targets Akt in host cells as an intracellular antiapoptotic strategy. Science Signaling. 2009;**2**:ra74. DOI: 10.1126/scisignal.2000374

[108] Manning BD, Cantley LC. AKT/PKB signaling: navigating downstream. Cell. 2007;**129**:1261-1274. DOI: 10.1016/jcell.2007.06.009.PMID:17604717

[109] Stahl P, Ruppert V, Meyer T, Campos MA, Gazzinelli RT, Maisch B, et al. Trypomastigotes and amastigotes of *Trypanosoma cruzi* induce apoptosis and STAT3 activation in cardiomyocytes in vitro. Apoptosis. 2013;**18**:653-663. DOI: 10.1007/s10495-013-0822-x

[110] Duaso J, Rojo G, Jaña F, Galanti N, Cabrera G, Bosco C, et al. *Trypanosoma cruzi* induces apoptosis in ex vivo infected human chorionic villi. Placenta. 2011;**32**:356-361. DOI: 10.1016/j.placenta.2011.02.005

[111] Morillo DA, González BE, Sulbarán AJ. La infección por *Trypanosoma cruzi* disminuye el desarrollo del melanoma maligno e incrementa la supervivencia en ratones C57BL/6. Investigación Clínica. 2014;**55**(3):227-237

[112] Urquiza JM, Burgos JM, Ojeda DS, Pascuale CA, Leguizamón MS, Quarleri JF. Astrocyte apoptosis and HIV replication are modulated in host cells coinfected with *Trypanosoma cruzi*. Frontiers in Cellular and Infection Microbiology. 2017;**7**:1-16. DOI: 10.3389/fcimb.2017.00345

Chapter 8

# Evaluation of Molecular Variability of Isolates of *Trypanosoma cruzi* in the State of Rio de Janeiro-Brazil

*Helena Keiko Toma, Luciana Reboredo de Oliveira da Silva, Teresa Cristina Monte Gonçalves, Renato da Silva Junior and Jacenir R. Santos-Mallet*

**Abstract**

*Trypanosoma cruzi*, the etiological agent of Chagas disease, presents considerable heterogeneity among populations of isolates within the sylvatic and domestic cycle. This study aims to evaluate the genetic diversity of 14 isolates collected from specimens of *Triatoma vitticeps* from Triunfo, Conceição de Macabu, and Santa Maria Madalena cities (Rio de Janeiro—Brazil). By using PCR based on the mini-exon gene, all isolates showed a profile characteristic of bands zymodeme III and with a lower intensity characteristic of TcII. To verify possible hybrids among the strains analyzed, the polymorphisms analysis of the MSH2 gene was performed. HhaI restriction enzyme digestion products resulted in characteristic TcII fragments only, demonstrating the absence of hybrids strains. In our attempt to characterize isolation in accordance with the reclassification of *T. cruzi* into six new groups called DTUs ("discrete typing unit"), we genotyped the mitochondrial cytochrome oxidase subunit two gene, ribosomal RNA gen (24Sα rDNA), and the spliced leader intergenic region (SL-IR). This procedure showed that TcII, TcIII, and TcIV are circulating in this area. This highlights the diversity of parasites infecting specimens of *T. vitticeps*, emphasizing the habit of wild type and complexity of the region epidemiological study that presents potential mixed populations.

**Keywords:** molecular biology, natural infection, triatomine, *Trypanosoma cruzi*, heterogeneity

## 1. Introduction

*Trypanosoma cruzi (T. cruzi)* is a heterogeneous parasite, in which strains are composed of different sub-populations or clones that circulate in nature between triatomine vectors, wild and domestic mammals, including man. The need for adaptation and survival in different hosts appears to be responsible for the high genetic diversity of the parasite [1] and the various clinical manifestations observed in Chagas' disease [2, 3].

The heterogeneity of strains of this parasite has been demonstrated using different markers: morphological, biological susceptibility to chemotherapeutic agents, immunological, biochemical and molecular [4–13].

Considerable advances have been made to understand the genetic makeup of *T. cruzi* and the process that involves the control of gene expression of the parasite. Molecular genetic markers have been used to correlate different strains with their different biological properties, clinical and epidemiological characteristics [14].

Ribosomal gene sequences have been widely used to infer phylogenetic relationships among the trypanosomatids and representatives of other families of the order Kinetoplastida and phylum Euglenozoa. In trypanosomes, the sequence of the 24S subunit is interrupted by an internal spacer generating two molecules, 24Sα and 24Sβ.

The conserved non-transcribed regions of the pre-rRNA correspond to the internal transcribed spacer (ITS) and external (ETS). The presence of several regions, transcribed or not, that display varying degrees of variability, entail a high degree of polymorphism of the ribosomal cistrons and for this reason, have proved to be excellent as a tool for identification and phylogenetic studies of trypanosomes [15]. The ITS spacers are highly variable compared with ITS which, in turn, are much more variable regions of the Small Sub Unit (SSU) and Large Sub Unit (LSU). Analysis of polymorphism of ribosomal sequences has been used in the identification and genotyping of strains.

Souto and cols. [16] standardized a marker based on the region of the LSU 24Sα, which distinguishes the *T. cruzi* I and *T. cruzi* II strains. Another excellent marker for the study of diversity in *T. cruzi* gene is the Mini-Exon. The identification of strains (genotyping) using PCR methods based on gene sequences of mini-exon has been widely used [16–20].

Due to its organization comprising regions with differing degrees of conservation of the mini-exon genes have been used for diagnosis purposes and taxonomic. Each repeating unit of the Spliced Leader (SL) gene can be basically divided into three parts: a highly conserved exon of 39 nucleotides, an intron moderately conserved nucleotides 50–100 and an intergenic spacer region, which varies in size and sequence among trypanosomes species and strains. There are about 200 repeated copies of the SL gene "in tandem" in the trypanosomes genome which are therefore a good target for diagnosis [21–23]. The use of PCR methods for genotyping based on the mini-exon and ribosomal genes segregates this parasite into three major lineages: *T. cruzi* I, *T. cruzi* II and Z3 [16, 20, 24].

Augusto-Pinto and cols [25] demonstrated that *T. cruzi* can be divided into three distinct haplogroups called A, B and C, based on an analysis of polymorphisms in the MSH2 gene of several strains of this parasite. It was subsequently found that strains of haplogroups B and C have a lower efficiency of the mismatching error repair (MMR) compared to strains of haplogroup A after treatment with cisplatin hydroxide and hydrogen [26].

These results suggested that the lower efficiency of MMR of haplogroups B and C could be associated with an increased generation of genetic variability in these strains. Thus an analysis of genetic variability by targeting the gene encoding the *T. cruzi* called TcAg48 is present in a large number of copies in the genome of this parasite. Digestion of the amplified product of a region of this gene with the restriction enzyme *Hha*I allowed by the group 35 strains in the same haplogroups already described for the analysis of MSH2. It was found even greater genetic variability of this antigen in strains belonging to haplogroups B and C, which showed a less efficient MMR. Some of the haplogroup B strains have a digestion pattern with characteristics of both strains of haplogroup B and C, indicating a hybrid character.

Zingales and cols [13] standardized nomenclature into six groups (*T. cruzi* I-VI), each group termed DTU ("discrete typing unit"), where DTU is defined by a set of strains that are genetically similar, and that can be identified by molecular markers common or immunological [27]; DTUs *T. cruzi* I and *T. cruzi* II respond to two groups originally defined at the first meeting [28]. Although it was evident that the V-VI DTUs correspond to hybrid organisms, their origin swims from different events of genetic exchange.

This study aimed to evaluate the genetic diversity of 14 isolates of specimens of *Triatoma vitticeps* collected from the locality of Triunfo, 2nd District of the municipality of Santa Maria Madalena and Conceição Macabu from Rio de Janeiro State.

## 2. Materials and methods, results and discussion

### 2.1 Parasites

The isolates were obtained from specimens of *Triatoma vitticeps* captured in the locality of Triunfo whose latitude is 22° 02′52″S and longitude 41° 56′ 32″W, in the Santa Maria Madalena and Conceição Macabu cities, both the State of Rio de Janeiro. In this study, we used a total of 14 samples obtained from triatomines collected in three distinct regions for this study called A, B and C. Six of them (SMM1, SMM10, SMM51, SMM57, SMM88 and SMM98) were isolated from area A, area deforested to make way for banana cultivation, being located at an altitude of 250 m and 3.5 km away from the village, seven samples (SMM9, SMM30, SMM34, SMM36, SMM39, SMM82 and SMM89) from area B, located in a valley with vegetation preserved around thinking to 130 m above sea level and 4 km far from the village. These two areas are 2 km far from each other and separated by mountainous area with altitudes between 400 and 900 m, belonging to the locality of Triunfo, Municipality of Santa Maria Madalena. One sample (SMM106) were isolated from D area, a preserved area of 10 km far from area C.

### 2.2 Growth of parasite

The samples were maintained in tubes containing NNN medium plus LIT (Liver Infusion Tryptose), as the liquid phase, supplemented 30% fetal calf serum. The tubes were incubated in an oven of the BOD (FANEM) to 27.3°C, subcultured regularly at intervals of 14 days for maintenance of the samples.

### 2.3 DNA extraction

Cultures of *T. cruzi* (10 ml) in the exponential growth phase were washed three times by centrifugation in PBS (Phosphate Buffered Saline) at 2,000 rpm for 10 minutes. After removal of the supernatant, the DNA was extracted by DNAzol (Invitrogen) following the manufactured instructions.

## 3. Polymerase chain reaction (PCR)

### 3.1 Mini-exon gene

The variability of the intergenic region of the gene of the mini-exon of the samples was studied using the technique of multiplex PCR, using primers TcI, TcII, Z3, Tr and ME [24]. These primers generate an amplification product of 200 bp (TcI), 250 bp (TcII), 150 bp (Z3) and 100 bp (*T. rangeli*). The reaction was conducted in a final volume for each sample of 50 μl containing ~100 ng of DNA template, 1U Taq Gold DNA polymerase (Invitrogen), 0.2mM of dNTPs, 1.5mM $MgCl_2$, buffer 1X (10mM Tris-HCl pH 8.5), 10 pmol of each primer (TcI, TcII, Z3, Tr and ME). Fragment amplification was carried out under the following temperature conditions: initial denaturation at 94°C/5 min and 5 cycles (94°C/1 min, 50°C/1 min, 72°C/1 min), followed by 25 cycles (94°C/30 sec, 55°C/30 sec, 72°C/30 sec) and a final extension at 72°C/5 min. Amplification products were analyzed by electrophoresis on 2.5% agarose gel and visualized under UV light after ethidium bromide staining. Dm 28c (TcI), CL Brener (TcII), 3663 (Z3) and R1625 (*Trypanosoma rangeli*) strains were used as control.

### 3.2 MSH2 gene

The study to check possible characters hybrids between the strains analyzed was made based on an analysis of the MSH2 gene polymorphisms with the digestion of the 875bp amplification product of a region of this gene with the restriction enzyme *Hha*I [26]. The reaction was conducted in a final volume for each sample of 50 μl containing ~100 ng of DNA template, 1U Taq DNA polymerase (Thermo Fisher Scientific), 0.2mM of dNTPs, 1.5mM $MgCl_2$, buffer 1X (10mM Tris-HCl pH 8.8, 50mM KCl, 0.8% Nonidet P40), 10 pmol of each primer (tmuts30 and tmuts41). PCR reaction was carried out under the following conditions: initial denaturation at 94°C/5 min and 30 cycles (94°C/30 sec, 55°C/1 min and 72°C/2 min). The fragment obtained by PCR was then digested with the *Hha*I restriction enzyme for 16 h at 37°C. The digestion products were analyzed by polyacrylamide gel electrophoresis in 7.5%. The gels were revealed by silver impregnation (DNA Silver Staining Kit /Amersham Biosciences).

### 3.3 Mitochondrial cytochrome oxidase subunit 2 (COII)

Polymorphism in mitochondrial cytochrome oxidase subunit 2 (COII) gene was analyzed using the Tcmit-10 and Tcmit-21 primers that amplified a fragment of approximately 375 bp [29]. The reaction was conducted in a final volume for each sample of 50 μl containing ~100 ng of DNA template, 1U Taq DNA polymerase (Thermo Fisher Scientific), 0.2mM of dNTPs, 1.5mM $MgCl_2$, buffer 1X (10mM Tris-HCl pH 8.8, 50mM KCl, 0.8% Nonidet P40), 10 pmol of each primer (tcmit10 and tcmit21). The reaction was performed under the following temperature conditions: 95°C/5 min and 40 cycles of 95°C/45 sec, 48°C/45 sec and 72°C/1 min and a final extension of 72°C/10 min. The obtained fragments were digested with *Alu*I restriction endonuclease and the polymorphism was analyzed after electrophoresis in 6.5% acrilamide gel. Dm28c (TcI), Y (TcII), 3663 (TcIII), 4167 (TcIV), (TcV) and CL Brener (TcVI) strains were used as control.

### 3.4 Ribosomal RNA gene (24Sα)

The study segment of the ribosomal RNA gene (DNAr24Sα) *T. cruzi* was performed using primers D71 and D72 [16]. These primers generate an amplification product of 110 bp and 125 bp for TcI to TcII, respectively. The reaction was conducted in a final volume for each sample of 50 μl containing ~100 ng of DNA template, 1U Taq DNA polymerase (Thermo Fisher Scientific), 0.2mM of dNTPs, 1.5mM $MgCl_2$, buffer 1X (10mM Tris-HCl pH 8.8, 50 mM KCl, 0.8% Nonidet P40), 10 pmol of each primer (D71 and D72).

Fragment amplification was carried out under the following temperature conditions: initial denaturation at 94°C/4 min and 30 cycles (94°C/1 min, 62.5°C/1 min, 72°C/1 min), followed by a final extension at 72°C/5 min. The visualization of the amplification product was performed by polyacrylamide gel electrophoresis in 7.5%. The gels were revealed by silver impregnation (DNA Silver Staining Kit/Amersham Biosciences). Dm28c (characterized as TcI) and CL Brener (characterized as TcII) strains were used as controls.

### 3.5 Spliced leader intergenic region (SL-IRac) gene

The amplification of the spliced intergenic region (SL-IRac) gene was realized with TcIII and UTCC primers in order to distinguish TcIII (fragment of 200 bp) and other DTU (fragment of 150 to 157 bp). The reaction was conducted in a final volume for each sample of 50 μl containing ~100 ng of DNA template, 1U Taq DNA polymerase (Thermo Fisher Scientific), 0,2mM of dNTPs, 1.5mM $MgCl_2$, buffer 1X (10mM Tris-HCl pH 8.8, 50mM KCl, 0.8% Nonidet P40), 10 pmol of each primer (TcIII and UTCC). The reaction was performed under the following temperature conditions: 95°C/5 min, 3 cycles of 94°C/30 sec, touch down 70–64°C/30 sec, 72°C/1 min and 33 cycles of 94°C/30 sec, 62°C/30 sec and 72°C/1 min and final extension of 72°C/10 min. The final products were visualized by electrophoresis in 6.5% acrylamide gel. Dm28c and 3663 strains were used as control.

## 4. Results

### 4.1 Variability of the intergenic region of the mini-exon gene

All 14 isolates of *T. cruzi* analyzed showed a band of 150 bp characteristic of the zymodeme III. Still in the same analysis also showed bands with a lower intensity of ~ 250pb characteristic of the group TcII, suggesting the presence of possible blends in the isolates (**Figure 1**).

### 4.2 Variability of the segment of ribosomal RNA gene (24Sα)

PCR amplification of ribosomal RNA gene (24Sα) using primers D71 and D72 resulted in fragments 125pb characteristic of lineage TcII (not shown).

### 4.3 MSH2 gene

The products of digestion with *Hha*I restriction enzyme resulted in fragments of 173pb, 207pb and 294pb for all isolates, which indicate a characteristic pattern for the TcII, so demonstrating that there is not possibly hybrids between our isolates (**Figure 2**).

### 4.4 DTU genotyping

DTU was determined according to D′Ávila *et al.* [30] that propose a three-step assay: polymorphism of the mitochondrial cytochrome oxidase subunit 2 (COII) after digestion with restriction enzyme *Alu*I (**Figure 3**), amplification of the D7 divergent domain of the 24Sα rRNA gene (**Figure 4**) and amplification of the spliced leader intergenic region (SL-IRac) (**Figure 5**).

According to the results, it was possible to determine DTU. Most of them showed the presence of two mixed *T. cruzi* populations (**Table 1**).

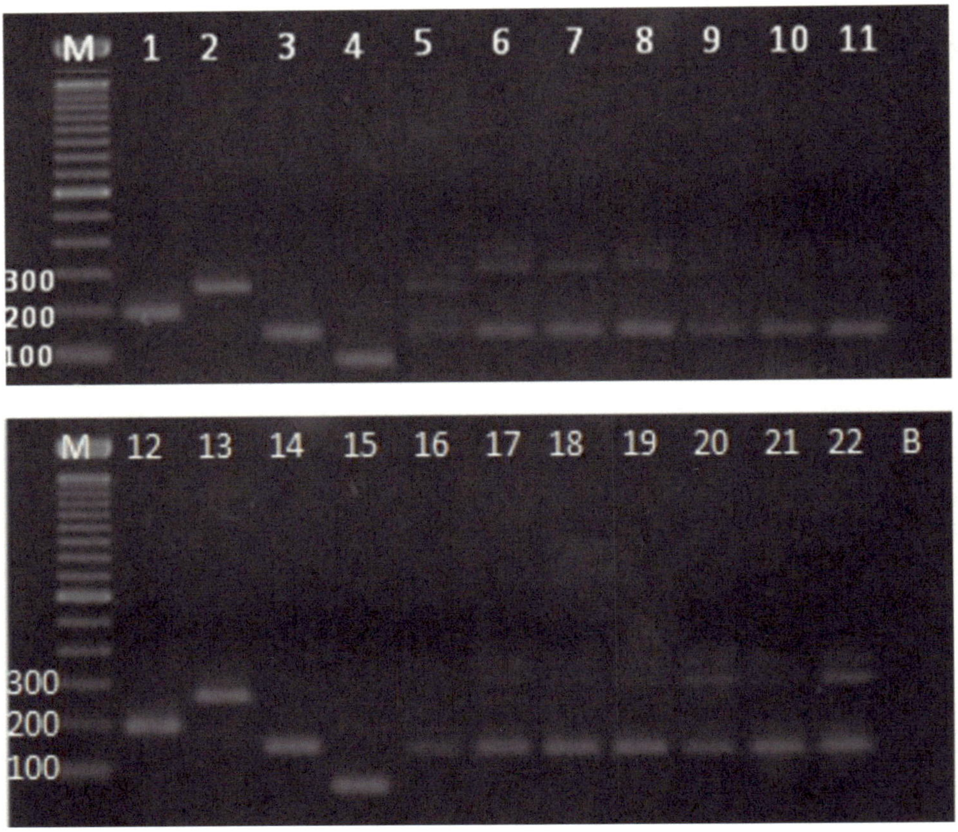


**Figure 1.**
*Molecular characterization of Trypanosoma cruzi isolates by segment analysis of the non-transcribed spacer of the mini-exon gene obtained by electrophoresis in agarose gel stained with ethidium bromide. M—molecular marker (100bp), lanes 1 and 12—control sample of Tc I (Dm 28c), 2 and 13—control sample of Tc II (CL Brener), 3 and 14—ZIII (3663), 4 and 15—control sample of T. rangeli (R1625), 5—SMM1, 6—SMM9, 7—SMM10, 8—SMM30, 9—SMM34, 10—SMM36, 11—SMM39. 16—SMM51, 17—SMM57, 18—SMM82, 19—SMM88, 20—SMM89, 21—SMM98, 22—SMM106, B—negative control.*

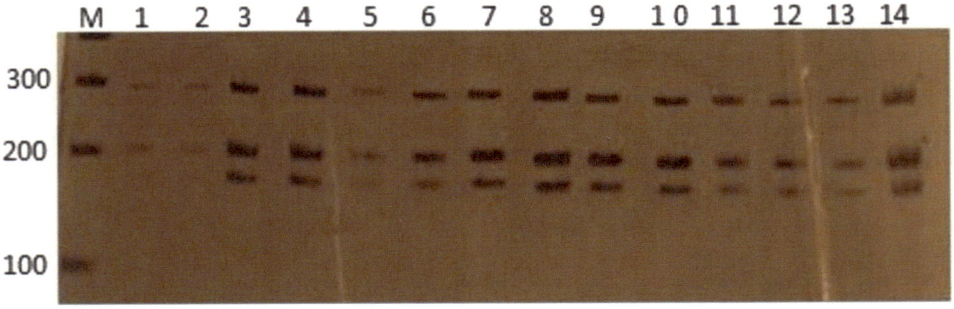


**Figure 2.**
*Electrophoresis in polyacrylamide Gel 7.5% of MSH2 gene after the restriction digestion enzyme HhaI. M—molecular marker (100 bp), 1—SMM1, 2—SMM9, 3—SMM10, 4—SMM30, 5—SMM34, 6—SMM36, 7—SMM39, 8—SMM51, 9—SMM57, 10—SMM82, 11—SMM88, 12—SMM89, 13—SMM98, 14—SMM106.*

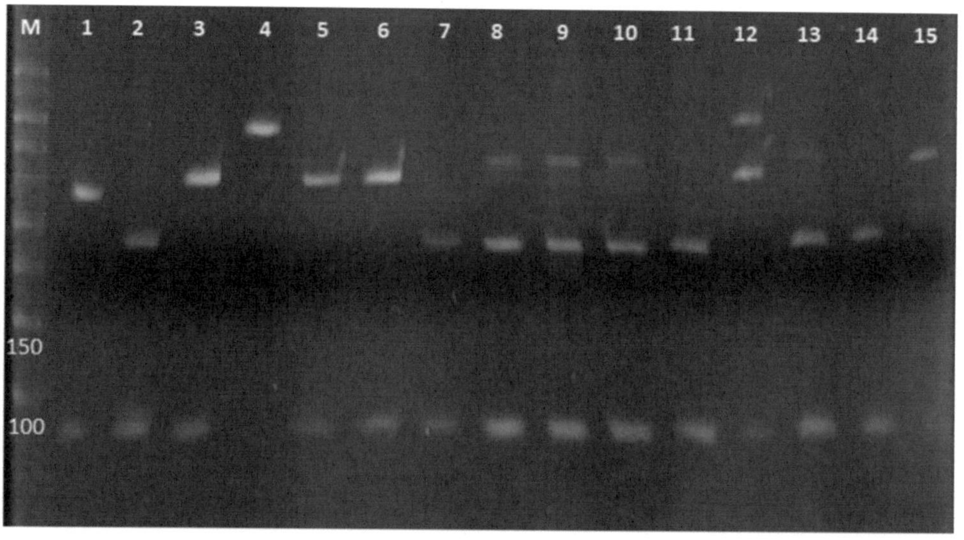


**Figure 3.**
*Electrophoresis in acrylamide gel of COII gene after digestion with AluI restriction enzyme. M—molecular marker (50 bp), 1–6—TcI-TcVI controls (1—haplotype A, 2—haplotype C, 3,5,6—haplotype B, 4—uncutted), 7–15 samples.*

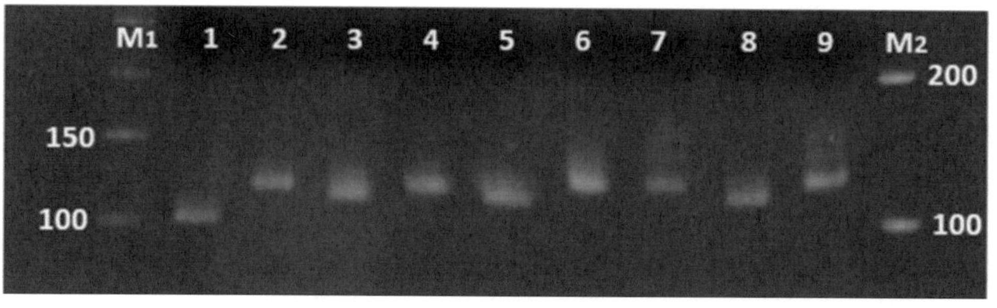


**Figure 4.**
*Electrophoresis in acrylamide gel of 24Sα gene. M1—molecular marker (50 bp), 1—TcI, 2—TcII, 3–9—samples, M2 molecular marker (100 bp).*

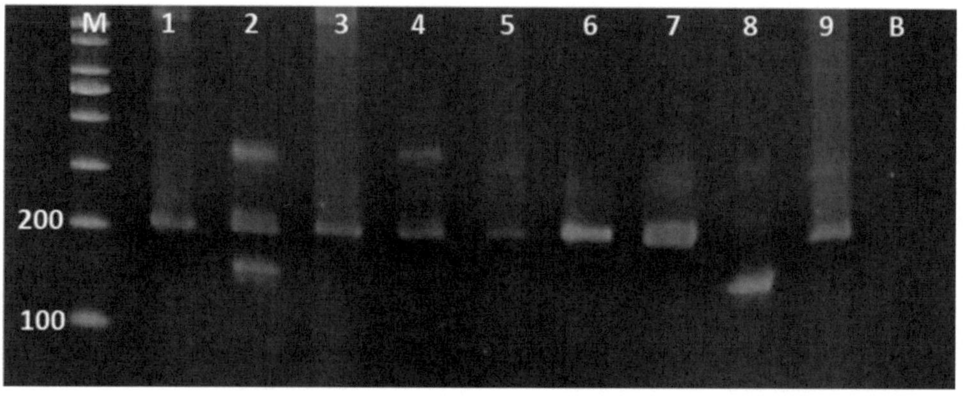


**Figure 5.**
*Electrophoresis in acrylamide gel of SL-IRac gene. M1—molecular marker (100 bp), 1–7—samples, 8 and 9—controls, B—negative control.*

| Cepa | Mini-Exon | Tcmit | 24S-rDNA | SL-IR | DTU |
|---|---|---|---|---|---|
| SMM1 | Z3 TcII | 212[a] | 125[a] | 150[a] | TcII[a] |
| SMM9 | Z3 TcII | 212[a], 294[b] | 125[a] | 200[b] | TcII[a], TcIV[b] |
| SMM11 | Z3 TcII | 212[a], 294[b] | 125[a] | 150[a], 200[b] | TcII[a], TcIV[b] |
| SMM30 | Z3 TcII | 212[a], 294[b] | 125[a] | 150[a], 200[b] | TcII[a], TcIV[b] |
| SMM34 | Z3 | 294 | 125 | 200 | TcIV |
| SMM36 | Z3 | 212[a], 294 | 117[b] | 150[a], 200[b] | TcII[a], TcIV[b] |
| SMM39 | Z3 | 212 | 125 | 150, (200) | TcII |
| SMM51 | Z3 | 294 | 125 | 200 | TcIV |
| SMM57 | Z3 TcII | 212[a], 294[b] | 125[a] | 150[a], 200[b] | TcII[a], TcIV[b] |
| SMM82 | Z3 TcII | 294 | 125 | 200 | TcIV |
| SMM88 | Z3 TcII | 212 | 125 | 150, (200) | TcII |
| SMM89 | Z3 TcII | 212 | 125 | 150, (200) | TcII |
| SMM98 | Z3 TcII | 294 | 125 | 200 | TcIV |
| SMM106 | Z3 TcII | 212 | 125 | (200) | TcII |

[a]*Compatible results with TcII.*
[b]*Compatible results with TcIV.*

**Table 1.**
*General results obtained in this work by the molecular characterization of isolates of* Trypanosoma cruzi *by different markers.*

## 5. Discussion

Many studies have been performed for the characterization of isolates of *Trypanosoma cruzi* obtained from human cases, animal reservoirs and triatomines mainly in Latin America, highlighting the heterogeneity of this species [31–39].

In previous studies using isoenzyme analysis, samples of zymodemes were grouped into three and were related to different isozyme groups found with the epidemiological profile of the isolates. Thus, zymodemes I (Z1) and III (Z3) are related to the sylvatic cycle of the parasite and zymodeme II (Z2) to the domestic cycle [7, 40]. Through molecular biology techniques [10, 12, 16, 20, 41–46] was able to evidence a clear dimorphism between the isolates of *T.cruzi*, leading to pooling of samples into two major phylogenetic lineages: Tc I and TcII. Related phylogenetic groups with TcI and TcII zymodemes: TcI was related to the Z1 and TcII be related to the Z2. However, the position of Z3 in relation to TcI and TcII phylogenetic groups remains controversial and is constantly debated. Some authors consider that Z3 is phylogenetically closer than TcI/TcII [19, 47, 48], while other authors consider the opposite [49–51]. However, other authors have included Z3 in an intermediate position between Z1 and Z2 [52].

In 2009 the scientific community was divided into six groups (Tc I-VI) and each group was termed DTU ("discrete typing unit"), which can be identified by the markers molecular or common immunological [27]. In the 70s and 80s, a large number of "group" was identified, and 90 years in 2000, only two major groups, and currently six groups.

In this study, samples of *T. cruzi* isolated from *Triatoma vitticeps* from the municipality of Santa Maria Magadalena, State of Rio de Janeiro, were analyzed by several molecular markers, showing a mixed population. The 14 isolates analyzed for the variability of the intergenic region of the Mini-Exon gene showed a profile of bands with 150 bp characteristic of zymodeme III and bands with a lower intensity with ~ 250pb, also indicating a profile for TcII. The PCR amplification of the ribosomal RNA gene (24Sα) using the primers D71 and D72 resulted in fragments 125pb showing a characteristic line TcII. In order to verify possible hybrid characters among the strains analyzed was done with PCR using specific primers tmuts30 and tmuts41 based on analysis of polymorphisms in the MSH2 gene with the digestion of the amplification product of a region of this gene with the restriction enzyme *Hha*I (*Haemophilus haemolyticus*) which resulted in fragments of 173pb, 207 pb and 294pb for each isolate, which also indicated a pattern characteristic for strain Tc II, showing then there is no hybrids between these isolates.

According to a protocol for determining DTU proposed by D´Ávila *et al.* [30] through the polymorphism analysis of the mitochondrial cytochrome oxidase subunit 2 (COII) gene, amplification of the D7 divergent domain of the 24Sα rRNA gene and amplification of the spliced leader intergenic region (SL-IRac) was possible to found two DTU circulating in the studied area.

Our results corroborate the hypothesis that isolated from *T. cruzi* infection may be a product of a mixture of populations of parasites as the vector into the wild environment can feed on various mammalian hosts. This complex was demonstrated by Fernandes *et al.* [18] in a study in the state of Rio de Janeiro showed that the association of two strains (TcI and TcII) with different wild hosts.

Evidence indicates that different populations of *T. cruzi* may circulate in nature by independent cycles of transmission and that these may, under certain conditions, if overlap. In these cases of overlapping cycles, one must admit that possibly different populations, which remained isolated, start to interact in the same vector and/or host. But while there is that possibility, little is known about these mechanisms between these different populations when they come into sympatry. The remarkable capacity of the parasite to infect several species implies adaptation of the parasite to live in various microhabitats, including the different segments of the intestinal tract of the insect [53, 54], nucleated mammalian cells including macrophages [55], blood and also the discharge of the scent glands some marsupials [56, 57]. Some of these are apparently microhabitats hostile to the development of the parasite [58].

Experimental studies have shown that mixed infection with *T. cruzi* can have a major impact on the biological properties of the parasite in the host, emphasizing the possible occurrence of natural mixed infections in humans and its consequences on the biological aspects of Chagas disease [2].

Our isolates showed indeed a correlation TcIV (formerly Z3) with TcII, indicating that these locality samples associating both the sylvatic cycle, as the domestic cycle, respectively, confirming the complexity of the sylvatic cycle of the disease. These results suggest that in this area might occur studied cycle *T. cruzi* epidemiological characteristics proposed by Zingales *et al.* [12], where both strains circulate in the wild habitat.

As TcV and TcVI, TcII has rarely been recorded in wild cycles and their natural niches are not well defined. Recent studies have demonstrated that TcII strain was isolated from opossums and primates in the wild forest, which led to the suggestion that primates could be the primary mammalian hosts of original TcII [59].

TcIV is relatively the more poorly understood group. It is the type responsible for the cause of Chagas disease in Venezuela [48] and was also responsible for the first record of an outbreak of acute cases simultaneously orally transmitted Chagas disease in the suburb of Canudos, State of Belém do Pará/Brazil [40].

Understanding the distribution and phylogeography of TcIV is complicated by the fact that several genotyping methods can not distinguish this strain from others, particularly TcIII.

It is important to emphasize that, TcIV and TcI is known to be endemic, in, North America, and were associated with raccoons in this region [60, 61]. Moreover, there is evidence that TcIV in North America is quite different from TcIV in South America [49, 62], and the presence of identical sequences of mitochondrial DNA in North America strains TcIV and TcI lineages suggests that genetic exchange has contributed to the diversity of strains seen in North America ([51]; Yeo *et al*, unpublished data).

The existence of mixed populations isolated from the *T. vitticeps* may reflect the pressure that these insects are suffering due to human action, prompting them to move into different ecological niches, increasing the possibility of contracting the infection of different hosts [63].

Genotyping demonstrates that the strains have a history that makes biological sense with widely current ecological structure, although the details are not yet well elucidated, but still require further research. The study of the genetic diversity of *T. cruzi* is of great importance for the control of Chagas disease. As seen, the application of molecular methods has shown that this parasite is possibly a body, but a fascinating complex heterogeneous, which will inevitably have different phenotypes. Molecular epidemiology can reveal the different types of transmission cycles and this is very important to develop strategies for vector control and understand their limitations.

## Author details

Helena Keiko Toma[1], Luciana Reboredo de Oliveira da Silva[2], Teresa Cristina Monte Gonçalves[3], Renato da Silva Junior[3,4] and Jacenir R. Santos-Mallet[3,5,6]*

1 Faculty of Pharmacy, Laboratory of Molecular Diagnosis and Hematology, Federal University of Rio de Janeiro-UFRJ, Rio de Janeiro, Brazil

2 Central Public Health Laboratory—LACEN-BA, Salvador, Brazil

3 Interdisciplinary Laboratory of Entomological Surveillance in Diptera and Hemiptera—LIVEDIH, Oswaldo Cruz Institute-IOC-Fiocruz, Rio de Janeiro, Brazil

4 Faculty of Medical Sciences of Maricá, Laboratory of Vector Insects, University of Vassouras (Campus Maricá), Brazil

5 Fiocruz-Piaui Regional Office, Teresina, Piauí, Brazil

6 Iguaçu University—UNIG, Nova Iguaçu, Brazil

*Address all correspondence to: jacenir@ioc.fiocruz.br

## References

[1] Silveira JF. Biologia Molecular do *Trypanosoma cruzi*. In: Brener Z, Andrade ZA e Barral-Netto M, editors. Trypanosoma cruzi e Doença de Chagas. Editora Guanabara Koogan, RJ: Segunda Edição; 2000. pp. 48-74

[2] Martins LP, Castanho RE, Casanova C, Caravelas DT, Frias GT, Ruas-Neto AL, et al. Rupestrian triatomines infected by Trypanosomatidae, collected in Quaraí, Rio Grande do Sul. Revista da Sociedade Brasileira de Medicina Tropical. 2006;**39**(2):198-202

[3] Stanaway JD, Roth G. The burden of Chagas disease: Estimates and challenges. Global Heart. 2015;**10**(3):139-144

[4] Brener Z. Intraspecific Variations in *Trypanosoma cruzi*: Two Types of Parasite Populations Presenting Distinct Characteristics. Vol. 347. Washington: PAHO, Sci Pub; 1977. pp. 11-21

[5] Filardi LS, Brener Z. Susceptibility and natural resistance of *Trypanosoma cruzi* strains to drugs used clinically in Chagas disease. Transactions of the Royal Society of Tropical Medicine and Hygiene. 1987;**81**:755-759

[6] Krettli A, Weisz-Carrington P, Nussenzweig RS. Membrane-bound antibodies to bloodstream *Trypanosoma cruzi* in mice: Strain differences in susceptibility to complement-mediated lysis. Clinical and Experimental Immunology. 1979;**37**:416-423

[7] Miles MA, Lanhan SM, De Souza AA, Povoa DG. Further enzymic characters of *Trypanosoma cruzi* and their evaluation for strain identification. Transactions of the Royal Society of Tropical Medicine and Hygiene. 1980;**74**:221-242

[8] Schelemper J, Avila CM, Coura JR, Brener Z. Course of infection and histopathological lesions in mice infected with seventeen *Trypanosoma cruzi* strains isolated from chronic patients. Revista da Sociedade Brasileira de Medicina Tropical. 1983;**16**(1):23-30

[9] Schlemper BR Jr, Ishida MM, Steindel M, Gargioni R. Tripomastigota muito largo como padrão 14. morfológico de cepas do *Trypanosoma cruzi* do extremo sul do Brasil. Memórias do Instituto Oswaldo Cruz. 1986;**81**:191-198

[10] Steindel M, Dias Neto E, Menezes CPL, Romanha AJ, Simpson AJG. Random amplified polymorphic DNA analysis of *Trypanosoma cruzi* strains. Molecular and Biochemical Parasitology. 1993;**60**:71-80

[11] Steindel M, Toma HK, Ishida MMI, Murta SMF, Pinto CJC, Grisard EC, et al. Biological and isoenzymatic characterization of *Trypanosoma cruzi* strains isolated from sylvatic reservoirs and vectors from the state of Santa Catarina, Southern Brazil. Acta Tropica. 1995;**60**:167-177

[12] Zingales B, Souto RP, Mangia RH, Lisboa CV, Campbell DA, Coura JR, et al. Molecular epidemiology of American trypanosomiasis in Brazil based on dimorphisms of rRNA and mini-exon gene sequence. International Journal for Parasitology. 1998;**28**:105-112

[13] Zingales B, Andrade SG, Briones MRS, Campbell DA, Chiari E, Fernandes O, et al. A new consensus for *Trypanosoma cruzi* intraspecific nomenclature: Second revision meeting recommends TcI to TcVI. Memórias do Instituto Oswaldo Cruz (Impresso). 2009;**104**:1051-1054

[14] Moncayo A, Ortiz Yanise MI. An update on Chagas disease (human American trypanosomiasis). Annals of Tropical Medicine and Parasitology. 2006;**100**:663-667

[15] Sogin ML, Elwood HJ, Gunderson JH. Evolutionary diversity of eukaryotic small-subunit rRNA genes. Proceedings of the National Academy of Science USA. 1986;**83**:1383-1387

[16] Souto RP, Fernandes O, Macedo AM, Campbell DA, Zingales B. DNA markers define two major phylogenetic lineages of *Trypanosoma cruzi*. Molecular and Biochemical Parasitology. 1996;**83**(2):141-152

[17] Brisse S, Verhoef J, Tibayrenc M. Characterisation of large and small subunit rRNA and mini-exon genes further supports the distinction of six *Trypanosoma cruzi* lineages. International Journal for Parasitology. 2001;**31**(11):1218-1226

[18] Fernandes O, Mangia RH, Lisboa CV, Pinho AP, Morel CM, Zingales B, et al. The complexity of the sylvatic cycle of *Trypanosoma cruzi* in Rio de Janeiro state (Brazil) revealed by the non-transcribed spacer of the mini-exon gene. Parasitology. 1999;**118**:161-166

[19] Fernandes O, Souto RP, Castro JA, Pereira JB, Fernandes NC, Junqueira AC, et al. Brazilian isolates of *Trypanosoma cruzi* from humans and triatomines classified into two lineages using mini-exon and ribosomal RNA sequences. The American Journal of Tropical Medicine and Hygiene. 1998b;**58**(6):807-811

[20] Fernandes O, Sturm NR, Derre R, Campbell DA. The mini-exon gene: A genetic marker for zymodeme III of *Trypanosoma cruzi*. Molecular and Biochemical Parasitology. 1998;**95**:129-133

[21] Agabian N. Trans splicing of nuclear pre-mRNAs. Cell. 1990;**61**:1157-1160

[22] Davis RE. Spliced Leader RNA trans splicing in Metazoa. Parasitology Today. 1996;**12**:33-40

[23] Donelson JE, Zeng W. A comparison of trans-RNA splicing in trypanosomes and nematodes. Parasitology Today. 1990;**6**:327-334

[24] Fernandes O, Santos SS, Cupolillo E, Mendonça B, Derre R, Junqueira AC, et al. A mini-exon multiplex polymerase chain reaction to distinguish the major groups of *Trypanosoma cruzi* and *T. rangeli* in the Brazilian Amazon. Transactions of the Royal Society of Tropical Medicine and Hygiene. 2001;**95**(1):97-99

[25] Augusto-Pinto L, Bartholomeu DC, Teixeira SM, Pena SD, Machado CR. Molecular cloning and characterization of the DNA mismatch repair gene class 2 from the *Trypanosoma cruzi*. Gene. 2001;**272**:323-333

[26] Augusto-Pinto L, Teixeira SM, Pena SD, Machado CR. Single-nucleotide polymorphisms of the *Trypanosoma cruzi* MSH2 gene support the existence of three phylogenetic lineages presenting differences in mismatch-repair efficiency. Genetics. 2003;**164**:117-126

[27] Tibayrenc M. Genetic epidemiology of parasitic protozoa and other infectious agents: The need for an integrated approach. International Journal for Parasitology. 1998;**28**:85-104

[28] Anonimous. Recommendations from a satellite meeting. Memórias do Instituto Oswaldo Cruz. 1999;**94** (Suppl. 1):429-432

[29] D'ávila DA, Gontijo ED, Lages-Silva E, WSF M, Chiari E, LMC

G. Random amplified polymorphic DNA profiles of *Trypanosoma cruzi* isolates from chagasic patients with different clinical forms. Parasitology Research. 2006;**98**:455-461

[30] D'ávila DA, Macedo AM, Valadares HMS, Gontijo ED, De Castro AM, Machado CR, et al. Probing population dynamics of *Trypanosoma cruzi* during progression of the chronic phase in chagasic patients. Journal of Clinical Microbiology. 2009;**47**(6):1718-1725

[31] Cardinal MV, Lauricella MA, Ceballos LA, Lanati L, Marcet PL, Levin MJ, et al. Molecular epidemiology of domestic and sylvatic *Trypanosoma cruzi* infection in rural northwestern Argentina. International Journal for Parasitology.2008;**38**(13):1533-1543

[32] Santos JP, Silva-Jr R, Ricardo-Silva AH, Verly T, Brito C, Evangelista BBC, et al. Assessing the entomo-epiemiological situation of Chagas disease in the rural communities in the state of Piauí, Brazilian semi-arid region. Transactions of the Royal Society of Tropical Medicine and Hygiene. 2020a;**114**(11):820-829

[33] Gonzalez J, Muñoz S, Ortiz S, Anacona D, Salgado S, Galleguillos M, et al. Biochemical, immunological, and biological characterization of *Trypanosoma cruzi* populations of the Andean north of Chile. Experimental Parasitology. 1995;**81**(1):125-135

[34] Martínez-Díaz RA, Escario JÁ, Nogal-Ruiz JJ, Barrio G. A biological characterization of *Trypanosoma cruzi* strains. Memórias do Instituto Oswaldo Cruz. 2001;**96**:53-59

[35] Mello DA, Borges MM, Chiarini LH. Growth and differentiation in vitro of *Trypanosoma cruzi* strains isolated from wild animals. Revista de Saúde Pública. 1980;**4**(4):569-581

[36] Pacheco RS, de Brito CM, Sarquis O, Pires MQ, Borges-Pereira J, Lima MM. Genetic heterogeneity in *Trypanosoma cruzi* strains from naturally infected triatomine vectors in northeastern Brazil: Epidemiological implications. Biochemical Genetics. 2005;**43**(9-10):519-530

[37] Sánchez-Guillén Mdel C, Bernabé C, Tibayrenc M, Zavala-Castro J, Totolhua JL, Méndez-López J, et al. *Trypanosoma cruzi* strains isolated from human, vector, and animal reservoir in the same endemic region in Mexico and typed as *T. cruzi I*, discrete typing unit 1 exhibit considerable biological diversity. Memórias do Instituto Oswaldo Cruz. 2006;**101**(6):585-590

[38] Santos JP, Silva-Jr R, Ricardo-Silva AH, Verly T, Brito C, Evangelista BBC, et al. Assessing the entomo-epiemiological situation of Chagas disease in the rural communities in the state of Piauí, Brazilian semi-arid region. Transactions of the Royal Society of Tropical Medicine and Hygiene. 2020b;**114**(11):820-829

[39] Silva CS. Estudo morfobiológico e histopatológico de amostras silvestres de *Trypanosoma cruzi* isoladas de *Triatoma vitticeps* (Stal, 1959) no estado do Rio de Janeiro. Dissertação de Mestrado, Universidade Federal Rural do Rio de Janeiro. p. 85

[40] Miles MA, Souza A, Povoa M, Shaw JJ, Lainson R, Toye PJ. Isozymic heterogeneity of *Trypanosoma cruzi* in the first autochthonous patients with Chagas' disease in Amazonian Brazil. Nature. 1978;**272**(5656):819-821

[41] Avila HA, Goncalves AM, Nehme NS, Morel CM, Simpson L.

Schizodeme analysis of *Trypanosoma cruzi* stocks from South and Central America by analysis of PCR-amplified minicircle variable region sequences. Molecular and Biochemical Parasitology. 1990;**42**(2):175-187

[42] Macedo AM, Martins MS, Chiari E, Pena SD. DNA fingerprinting of *Trypanosoma cruzi*: A new tool for characterization of strains and clones. Molecular and Biochemical Parasitology. 1992;**55**:147-153

[43] Morel CM, Deane MP, Gonçalves AM. The complexity of *Trypanosoma cruzi* populations revealed by schizodeme analysis. Parasitology Today. 1986;*2*(*4*):97-101

[44] Mormori T. Characterization of *Trypanosoma cruzi* isolates, using restriction enzyme analysis of kinetoplast DNA. Nippon Rinsho. 1992;**50**(Suppl):475-479

[45] Tibayrenc M, Neubauer K, Barnabe C, Guerrini F, Skarecky D, Ayala FJ. Genetic characterization of six parasitic protozoa: Parity between random-primer DNA typing and multilocus enzyme electrophoresis. Proceedings of the National Academy of Science USA. 1993;**90**:1335-1339

[46] Vago AR, Macedo AM, Oliveria RP, Andrade LO, Chiare E, Galvao LM, et al. Kinetoplast DNA signatures of *Trypanosoma cruzi* strains obtained directy from infected tissues. The American Journal of Pathology. 1996;**149**:2153-2159

[47] Brandão A, Fernandes O. *Trypanosoma cruzi*: Mutation in the 3′ untranslated region of calmodulin gene are specific for lineages *T. cruzi* I, *T. cruzi* II, and Zymodema III isolates. Experimental Parasitology. 2006;**112**(4):247-252

[48] Miles MA, Povoa MM, Prata A, Cedilos RA, De Souza AA, Macedo V. Do radically dissimilar *Trypanosma cruzi* strains (zimodemes) cause Venezuelan and Brazilian forms of Chagas'disease? Lancet. 1981;**1**:1338-1340

[49] Barnabé C, Brisse S, Tibayrenc M. Population structure and genetic epidemiology of *Trypanosoma cruzi*, the agent of Chagas' disease: A multilocus enzyme electrophoresis approach. Parasitology. 2000;**120**:513-526

[50] Brisse S, Barnabé C, Tibayrenc M. Identification of six *Trypanosoma cruzi* phylogenetic lineages by random amplified polymorphic DNA and multilocus enzyme electrophoresis. International Journal for Parasitology. 2000;**30**:35-44

[51] Machado CA, Ayala FJ. Nucleotide sequences provide evidence of genetic exchange among distantly related lineages of *Trypanosoma cruzi*. Proceedings of the National Academy of Science USA. 2001;**98**:7396-7401

[52] Stothard JR, Frame IA, Carrasco HJ, Miles MA. On the molecular taxonomy of *Trypanosoma cruzi* using riboprinting. Parasitology. 1998;**117**:243-247

[53] Dias E. Estudos sobre o Schyzotrypanum cruzi. Memórias do Instituto Oswaldo Cruz. 1934;**28**:1-110

[54] Schaub GA, Boker CA. Colonization of the rectum of *Triatoma infestans* by *Trypanosoma cruzi*: Influence of the starvation studied by scanning electron microscopy. Acta Tropica. 1987;**43**:349-354

[55] Nogueira N, Cohn Z. *Trypanosoma cruzi*: Mechanism of entry and intracellular fate in mammalian cells. The Journal of Experimental Medicine. 1976;**143**(6):1402-1420

[56] Deane MP, Lenzi HL, Jansen A. *Trypanosoma cruzi*: Vertebrate and invertebrate cycles in the same mammal host, the opossum Didelphis marsupialis. Memórias do Instituto Oswaldo Cruz. 1984;**79**(4):513-515

[57] Steindel M, Pinto CJ. *Trypanosoma cruzi* development in the anal glands of experimentally infected *Lutreolina crassicaudata* (Marsupialia, Didelphidae). Memórias do Instituto Oswaldo Cruz. 1988;**83**(3):397

[58] Garcia ES, Azambuja P. Development and interactions of *Trypanosoma cruzi* in insect vector. Parasitology Today. 1991;7(9):240-244

[59] Lisboa CV, Mangia RH, de Lima NR, Martins A, Dietz J, Baker AJ, et al. Distinct patterns of *Trypanosoma cruzi* infection in Leonto-pithecus rosalia in distinct Atlantic Coastal Rainforest fragments in Rio de Janeiro, Brazil. Parasitology. 2004;**129**:703-711

[60] Clark CG, Pung OJ. Host specificity of ribosomal DNA variation in sylvatic *Trypanosoma cruzi* from North America. Molecular and Biochemical Parasitology. 1994;**66**:175-179

[61] Roellig DM, Brown EL, Barnabé C, Tibayrenc M, Steurer FJ, Yabsley MJ. Molecular typing of *Trypanosoma cruzi* isolates, United States. Emerging Infectious Diseases. 2008;**14**:1123-1125

[62] Marcili A, Lima L, Valente VC, Valente SA, Batista JS, Junqueira AC, et al. Comparative phylogeography of *Trypanosoma cruzi* TCIIc: New hosts, association with terrestrial ecotopes, and spatial clustering. Infection, Genetics and Evolution. 2009;**9**(6):1265-1274

[63] Gonçalves TCM, Oliveira E, Dias LS, Almeida MD, Nogueira WO, Ávila-Pires FD. An investigation on the ecology of *Triatoma vitticeps* (Stal, 1859) and its possible role in the transmission of *Trypanosoma cruzi*, in the locality of Triunfo, Santa Maria Madalena municipal district, state of Rio de Janeiro, Brasil. Memórias do Instituto Oswaldo Cruz. 1998;**93**:711-717